ALTERNATIVE CROPS AND CROPPING SYSTEMS

Edited by **Petr Konvalina**

Alternative Crops and Cropping Systems

http://dx.doi.org/10.5772/61408
Edited by Petr Konvalina

Contributors

Jestinos Mzezewa, Eastonce T Gwata, Andrew Price, Lina Sarunaite, Maciej Bosiacki, Bartosz Markiewicz, Tomasz Kleiber, Hussein Shimelis, Prince Matova, Jesús Alberto Vázquez-Rodríguez, Carlos Abel Amaya-Guerra, Petra Hlasna Cepkova, Dagmar Janovská, Jiří Hermuth, Zdislava Dvořáková, Sergej Usťak, Zdeněk Strašil, Leo Aoi Hosoya, Hajime Araki

CBS, Edition **2017**

Published by InTech

Janeza Trdine 9, 51000 Rijeka, Croatia

Publishing Process Manager Dajana Pemac

Technical Editor InTech DTP team

Cover Designer InTech Design Team

Additional hard copies can be obtained from orders@intechopen.com

Alternative Crops and Cropping Systems, Edited by Petr Konvalina
p. cm.
ISBN 978-953-51-2279-1

INTECH

open science | open minds

Contents

Contents

Preface

Alternative crops are cultural as well as newly bred crop species that replace, extend and complement the existing range of crops and contribute to broaden the spectrum of plant production. Basically, it is either a reintroduction of crops that have been previously cultivated but which, due to lower yields, quality, changes in technology or dietary habits was their cultivation reduced or discontinued altogether (e.g., Sorghum). The second group is the newly introduced crops – this is the second successful economic exploitation in other areas of the world. The main advantages of alternative crops include increased food diversity, but also the expansion of market opportunities for farmers.

Alternative cropping systems may represent an innovative approach to growing certain crops. General aim is to use different approach for the production of high quality of food. Approaches to growing plants may be different. It could be to minimize the negative impact of farming on the environment. On the other hand, it may be highly sophisticated system of cultivation such as hydroponics.

The book contains eight chapters written by acknowledged experts, providing comprehensive information on all aspects of alternative crops and cropping systems. The book is divided into two parts: alternative crops and alternative cropping systems. In the book there are chapters oriented towards sorghum and ulva growing and use. In the second part, there are chapters oriented to tomato production, rice production or herbicide and cover crop residue integration. Researchers, teachers and students in the agricultural field, in particular, will find this book to be of immense use.

The goal was to write a book where as many different existing studies as possible could be presented in a single volume, making it easy for the reader to compare methods, results and conclusions. As a result, studies from countries such as South Africa, Zimbabwe, Poland, The Czech Republic, Mexico and Japan have been compiled into one book. I believe that the opportunity to compare results and conclusions from different countries and continents will create a new perspective in alternative crops and cropping systems. I hope that our book will help researchers and students all over the world to attain new and interesting results in the field of alternative crops and cropping systems.

Dr. Petr Konvalina
Faculty of Agriculture
University of South Bohemia in České Budějovice
České Budějovice
Czech Republic

Section 1

Alternative Crops

Chapter 1

Sorghum and Foxtail Millet—Promising Crops for the Changing Climate in Central Europe

Jiří Hermuth, Dagmar Janovská,
Petra Hlásná Čepková, Sergej Usťak,
Zdeněk Strašil and Zdislava Dvořáková

Additional information is available at the end of the chapter

http://dx.doi.org/10.5772/62642

Abstract

Climate change is connected to many undesirable aspects which may strongly affect agricultural production in the future, not only in the Czech Republic but also in other countries in Central Europe. The most serious risks with the main impacts on agricultural production are the frequency and intensity of occurrence of extreme events. Problems caused by drought and its impact on agricultural production are starting to be serious and urgent. One of the solutions is using the drought-tolerant/resistant species and/or varieties more adaptable to water stress. Sorghum and foxtail millet might be the solution for Czech conditions. They can provide good yields even in dry periods. This study discusses grain quality of foxtail millet and biomass quality in the case of sorghum. In addition, the benefits of cultivation of these two species and current knowledge from a scientific point of view are summarised here.

Keywords: sorghum, foxtail millet, genetic resources, alternative crops, biomass production

1. Current situation

Climate change is connected to many undesirable aspects which may strongly affect agricultural production in the future, not only in the Czech Republic but also in other countries in Central Europe. The main signs of these changes are a lack of water, extreme fluctuation of weather, movement of vegetation, and floods. The most serious risks are then the frequency and intensity of occurrence of extreme events. The main impacts on agricultural production are declines in yield, increased crop failure, change in the geographical distribution of some plant species, the occurrence of invasive species, thermophilic diseases and pests, etc. Problems caused by drought and its impact on agricultural production are starting to be serious and urgent. In the Czech Republic, the most outstanding period of drought was recorded in 2012. In the region of South Moravia (part of the Czech Republic), the yield of winter wheat was lower by 22.8% in comparison with 2011. Czech agriculture faced a similar situation in 2015. Because these situations may repeat in the future as well, the Agrarian Chamber of the Czech Republic and the Ministry of Agriculture issued a recommendation and long-term system actions leading to the involvement of the state in solving these situations in the future. One of the recommendations is using non-technical measures, such as breeding and selection of drought resistant species and varieties more adaptable to water stress and more resistant to changing climate conditions.

Sorghum and foxtail millet might be the solution for Czech conditions. Research on the suitability of both mentioned species in the Czech Republic has been carried out at the Crop Research Institute (CRI) since the 1990s. The main aim is to evaluate and select suitable genotypes of sorghum and foxtail millet for human consumption, which may be an alternative to grain and for biomass production for arid areas of the Czech Republic as well as other countries in Central Europe. Both of these crops belong to the C4 species, which can better manage water through photosynthesis. They can provide good yields even in dry periods. This study discusses grain quality of foxtail millet and biomass quality in the case of sorghum. In addition, the benefits of cultivation of these two species and current knowledge from a scientific point of view are summarised here.

The group of millets refers to a number of different species such as *Panicum miliaceum* L., *Pennisetum glaucum* (L.) R.Br., *Setaria italica* (L.) P. Beauv. [1] early together with sorghum (*Sorghum bicolor* L.), and even maize (*Zea mays* L.). Millets and sorghum belong to the oldest cultivated crops, which have been very important staples and ethnobotanical crops in the semi-arid tropics of Asia and Africa for centuries [2, 3]. The millets and sorghum are various grass crops that are harvested for human food, animal feed, and medicinal purposes [4]. Sorghum is the fifth most important cereal in the world after wheat, rice, maize, and barley. Some 49 and 55% of the world's millet and sorghum cultivation areas, respectively, are in Africa. In India, millet is said to constitute the fourth most commonly grown cereal, following rice, wheat, and sorghum [5]. Although sorghum and millets account for about the same total production as maize, they account for nearly twice the cultivated area [1].

Foxtail millet and sorghum are high energy [6], nutritionally equivalent or superior to other cereals [7], and do not contain gluten-forming proteins. Sorghum is also a potentially important source of nutraceuticals such as antioxidants, phenolics, and cholesterol-lowering waxes [8]. Foxtail millet and sorghum play a significant role in food security for developing countries in Asia and Africa and also play a growing role in processing and new alternative products for the developed world [7]. They are of value especially in semiarid regions because of their short growing season and higher productivity under conditions where another cereal crops may fail [9]. Compared to other cereals, millets are mainly suited to less fertile soils and poorer growing conditions, such as intense heat and low rainfall [4, 9].

2. Introduction

2.1. Foxtail millet

Foxtail millet [*Setaria italica* (L.) P. Beauv.] is one of the oldest cereals in Eurasia [10], grown since 5000 BC in China and 3000 BC in Europe. It probably evolved from the wild green foxtail millet—*Setaria viridis* (L.) P. Beauv. [11–13]. The geographical origin of foxtail millet is still a controversial issue [14]. Its domestication could have taken place anywhere across its natural range extending from Europe to Japan, perhaps even several times independently; it was most probably first domesticated in the highlands of central China, from where it spread to India and Europe soon thereafter [11, 15]. At present, foxtail millet is cultivated all over the world, being most important in China, India, Indonesia, the Korean peninsula and south-eastern Europe [16]. In most countries in the world, foxtail millet is cultivated mainly for production of grains for human consumption. The tiny grains are milled into flour used for preparation of different dishes (puree, cakes, etc.). In China, Korea, and Japan, foxtail millet is important for beer preparation, with the sprouted seeds used instead of malt. Thanks to fermentation, various alcoholic beverages are prepared [17]. In Europe, seeds of foxtail millet are used for poultry feeding and plants are cultivated as a fodder crop for green biomass or hay production.

2.2. Sorghum

The greatest diversity in both cultivated and wild types of *Sorghum* Moench is found in north-eastern tropical Africa. It is thought that the crop was domesticated in Ethiopia by selection from wild sorghum types between 5000 and 7000 years ago [18]. Doggett [19] also considered Ethiopia and the surrounding countries as a centre of domestication. From north-eastern Africa, sorghum was probably distributed all over Africa and along shipping and trade routes through the Middle East to India [20]. Sorghum probably travelled overland from India and reached China [9] and South-East Asia [20] along the silk route about 2000 years ago. It might also have gone by sea directly from Africa. Chinese seamen reached Africa's east coast more than 1000 years ago (probably in the eighth century AD), and they may well have carried some seeds home [9]. From West Africa, sorghum was taken to the Americas through the slave trade. It was introduced into North America for commercial cultivation from North Africa, South Africa, and India at the end of the nineteenth century [20]. It was subsequently introduced into South America and Australia, where it has become an established grain and fodder crop. It is now widely cultivated in drier areas of Africa, Asia, the Americas, Europe (France, Italy, and Hungary) as well as Australia, Russia, and Argentina. It is cultivated between 50°N and 30°S latitude and up to 2200 m above sea level [16, 18]. Sorghum types exclusively cultivated for the dye in the leaf sheaths can be found from Senegal to Sudan [20]. Sorghum was introduced to the Czech Republic in the 1920s when it was used mainly as a fodder crop. Until 1950, the area of cultivated sorghum was higher than the introduced new maize varieties. In the first decade of the twenty-first century, the higher interest in sorghum cultivation is connected with the development of renewable energy for power plant feeding by biomass production due to the fact that sorghum provides it in high quality and amount.

3. Morphology

3.1. Foxtail millet

Foxtail millet is an erect annual grass [11], between 0.6 and 1.2 m tall, tufted, often variously tinged with purple. Its root system is dense, with thin wiry adventitious roots from the lowest nodes [15] (**Figure 1**).

The stem is erect, slender, tillering from the lower buds, sometimes branched. Primitive cultivars have numerous, strongly branched stems, while advanced cultivars produce a single stem with a large, solitary inflorescence [11].

Its leaves are alternate, simple [11]; leaf sheath cylindrical, 10–15 (−26) cm long, glabrous or slightly hairy; ligule short, fimbriate; blade linear-acuminate, 16–32 (−50) × 1.5–2.5(−4) cm, midrib prominent [15], slightly rough [11].

The inflorescence is a spike-like panicle 5–30 × 1–2(−5) cm, erect or pendulous, continuous or interrupted at the base; the rachis is ribbed and hairy; the lateral branches are short, bearing 6–12 spikelets. The spikelets are almost sessile, subtended by 1–3 bristles up to 1.5 cm long, elliptical, usually about half as long as the bristles [11].

Its fruit is a caryopsis (grain) [11], which is enclosed in coloured hulls [11, 21, 22] with the colour depending on the variety [21]. The grain is broadly ovoid, up to 2 mm long [11]. The colour of the grain varies from pale yellow to orange, red, brown, or black [23]. Generally, foxtail millet seeds are not dormant [24]. The 1000-seed weight is about 2 g [23].

Foxtail millet has a short vegetation crop [24]; total crop duration is 80–120 days, although some cultivars only need 60 days to mature [11]. Foxtail millet is largely self-pollinating with an average outcrossing rate of 4%; natural hybrids between wild and cultivated types occur. Foxtail millet has largely lost the ability of natural seed dispersal and shows a tendency toward uniform plant maturity [11].

3.2. Sorghum

Sorghum comes in many types. All, however, are coarse, cane-like grasses between 0.5 and 6 m tall [9], depending on the variety and growing conditions [25]. Most are annuals; a few are perennials [9]. Its roots are concentrated in the top 90 cm of the soil but sometimes extending to twice that depth, spreading laterally up to 1.5 m [9, 20].

The stem (culm) is solid [20], or sometimes with spaces in pith [26], usually erect [9, 20], 5–30 mm in diameter [25]. Stems may be dry or juicy. The juice may be either insipid or sweet. Most have a single stem, but some varieties tiller profusely, sometimes putting up more than a dozen stems. These extra stems may be produced early or late in the season [9].

The leaves are alternate, simple [20], broad and coarse, looking much like those of maize [9] but are shorter and wider [25]. A single plant may have as few as 7 or as many as 24 leaves, depending on the cultivar [9]. At first they are erect, but later curve downward. During drought, they roll their edges together. Rows of 'motor cells' in the leaves cause the rolling

http://dx.doi.org/10.5772/62642

action and provide this unusual method of reducing desiccation [9]. The leaf sheath is 15–35 cm long [20], often with a waxy bloom [27], with a band of short white hairs at the base near attachment, reddish in dye cultivars [20]. The leaf blade is lanceolate to linear-lanceolate, 30–135 cm long and 1.5–13.0 cm broad, initially erect, later curving, margins flat, or wavy [18].

The inflorescence is a terminal [20], more or less open panicle [28] (**Figure 2**), up to 60 cm long [20] and 5–25 cm broad [28]; the rachis is short or long, with primary, secondary, and sometimes tertiary branches, with spikelets in pairs and in groups of three at the ends of the branches [20]. Sorghum is predominantly self-pollinating [20].

The fruit is a caryopsis (grain) [20], typically thought of as round [29]. Due to the genetic diversity of sorghum, grains can vary widely in size and shape. Commercial sorghum hybrids are 4–8 mm long [20, 30], 2 mm broad [30], smaller than those of maize but with a similar starchy endosperm [9]. The grains are usually partially covered by glumes [20]; the seed coat varies in colour [9] from white [25], pale yellow through to red, purple-brown. Dark-coloured types generally taste bitter because of the tannins in the seed coat [9]. The 1000-seed weight varies from 13 to 80 g [20, 27, 30].

In the tropics and subtropics, sorghum may be one of the quickest maturing food plants [9]. Early maturing sorghum cultivars take only 100 days or less [20] and can provide three harvests a year [9], whereas in temperate areas it requires 5–7 months [20].

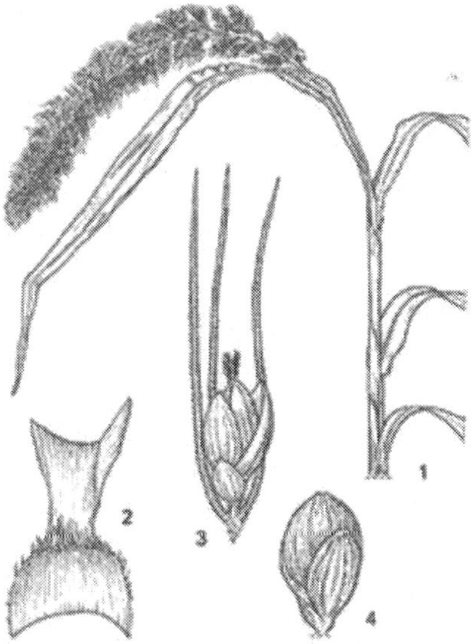

Figure 1. *Setaria italica* [11].

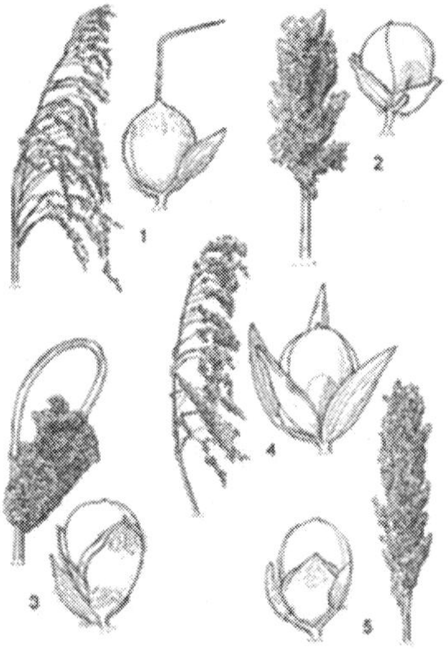

Figure 2. Panicles and spikelets of the 5 basic races of sorghum: 1—bicolor; 2—caudatum; 3—durra; 4—guinea; 5—kafir [18].

4. Breeding

4.1. Foxtail millet

Wang et al. [31] wrote the first mention of foxtail millet suitability for genetic and molecular studies due to the small genome size and its diploid nature. Genetic variability studies for the identification of trait-specific germplasm accessions for various agronomic and nutritional traits are lacking in foxtail millet, and are hence seldom used in breeding [32]. The major breeding objectives of foxtail millet are developing high-yielding cultivars which produce protein-rich seed and are resistant to diseases, pests, and lodging [33], and are adapted to local ecological conditions [15]. One of the important components of plant breeding programmes has been crop improvement through the introduction of novel genes from wild relatives [31, 34] with the research focused on salt stress responses in foxtail millet seedlings. In the Czech Republic, the breeding of foxtail millet accessions is performed by the Gene Bank of the CRI. The collection of foxtail millet includes 42 accessions in an active collection and 150 genotypes in a working collection. The main aim is to find foxtail millet genotypes as a new source of gluten-free grain, a source of feed for animals (hay and seeds) as well as for biomass production used in power plants. Based on the work with genetic resources of foxtail millet, a broad set of foxtail genotypes were chosen which were further selected (**Table 1**). The main sources of new genotypes are other gene banks, universities, or botanical gardens all over the world. Because some foxtail millet genotypes may be sensitive to daylight duration, the sensitivity to the day length is the main parameter of the evaluation. During the vegetation, several morphophenological characteristics and health assessment of plants were done. After harvest, all genotypes unsuitable for the temperate conditions of the Czech Republic were excluded from the collection. The evaluation was focused on the early-ripening genotypes, on the size of grains, as well as on production of high amount of biomass described by the plant height. In 2014, a new perspective variety of *Setaria italica* 'Ruberit' was bred in the Czech Republic suitable for the production of biomass, human consumption (corn), and livestock nutrition (grain and forage) (**Appendix I**) New genotype of *Setaria italica* 'Rucereus' bred for conditions of the Central Europe. Is now under testing of Central Institute for Supervising and Testing in Agriculture (**Appendix II**).

Year	New cultivated genotypes	Not grown up genotypes	Not flowering genotypes	Not ripening genotypes	Total no. of sown genotypes
2010	31 (37.8%)	0 (0%)	26 (31.7%)	25 (30.5%)	82 (100%)
2011	86 (86%)	0 (0%)	2 (2%)	12 (12%)	100 (100%)

Table 1. Summary of evaluation of new genetic resources of foxtail millet in the CRI, Prague Ruzyně.

4.2. Sorghum

To date, in the EU, there are 462 varieties of *Sorghum bicolor* registered. However, landraces and wild related species of sorghum are an important source of various properties for breeding, such as tolerance and resistance to pests and diseases, abiotic stresses such as lack of water and high temperature, as well as quality and nutrition content for feed, food, and technical utilisation [35]. Globally, in different gene banks, there are about 168,000 accessions of sorghum. In the USA, genetic resources from gene banks are used to create new lines of A-, B-, and R-, which then are used by private breeding companies producing new hybrid varieties. This shows the key role of the interconnection of private and public sector in the creation of new varieties [36]. To date, the International Union for the Protection of New Varieties of Plants (UPOV) has registered a total of 3951 varieties of *Sorghum bicolor* worldwide.

Sorghum is a short-day plant which uses the C4 photosynthesis system. Maturity is influenced by the length of day and temperature. Breeding starts with adapting short-day crop to conditions of the temperate zone to a longer day, and shortening the stalks for improved mechanical harvesting [36]. The most used techniques for breeding sorghum are the same as in the case of maize. Since the 1950s, the cytoplasmic male sterility (CMS) method has been used (**Table 2**).

The main objectives in sorghum breeding worldwide include high grain yield [37], resistance to major yield-limiting diseases and pests [38], drought tolerance [39–41], cold tolerance [42], and tolerance to the other abiotic stresses [43, 44]. Resistance to grain moulds [45, 46] and other diseases [20, 35, 47] as well as to insect pests [48] has been identified.

Line	Cytoplasm	Genotype	Phenotype
A-line	A	rfrf	Male sterility
B-line	N	rfrf	Male fertility
R-line	A or N	RFRF	Male fertility
Hybrid	A	RFrf	Male fertility

Table 2. Genotype and phenotype for A-, B-, and R-line in system of cytoplasmatic male sterility in; N—normal cytoplasm, A—sterility inducing by cytoplasmic [36].

In the northern part of Europe, the cultivation of sorghum has a certain tradition. In recent years, due to changing climate, sorghum cultivation has become attractive in the Central parts of Europe (Germany, Hungary, and Austria). The cultivated areas have increased and the breeding programmes of sorghum were established. They are bred for cold resistance, earliness, and decrease of anti-nutritional components in seeds [49]. It is necessary at the outset to state that a breeding programme for sorghum in the Czech Republic currently does not take place; we are merely introducing materials from countries where sorghum breeding programmes are supported.

When we select varieties of grain sorghum, those with the shortest growing season are chosen. Furthermore, a very important feature is the grain chemical composition. When grain is used for human food, the grain shape and size are important. Grain for food purposes may be depreciated and reduce the possibility of its use as a food due to high tannin content. Therefore, one of the important objectives in the context of grain sorghum breeding is to obtain these materials without anti-nutritional components. A very important role in breeding is played by the height of genotypes; the lower growth facilitates the process of mechanised harvesting. The Gene Bank of the CRI evaluated and selected potentially suitable genotypes for conditions in the Czech Republic. The plant material is mainly obtained from other world institutions, such as gene banks, universities, and botanical gardens, mainly from Europe, the USA, Australia, and countries in Asia. Several genotypes are obtained from private subjects. The plant material does not have characters of hybrids. All new accessions are tested over three successive years. Subsequently, original data are obtained showing suitability for applications of new plant materials in the conditions of the Czech Republic. These sorghum genotypes are described and stored in a gene bank under defined conditions as an important source of valuable genetic material for a potential breeding programme in the region of Central Europe.

Year	New cultivated genotypes	Not grown up genotypes	Not flowering genotypes	Not ripening genotypes	Total no. of sown genotypes
2010	59 (34.8%)	38 (22.3%)	7 (4.1%)	66 (38.8%)	170 (100%)
2011	58 (38.4%)	7 (4.6 %)	8 (5.3%)	78 (51.7%)	151 (100%)

Table 3. Summary of grain sorghum at the CRI, Prague Ruzyně.

The summary (**Table 3**) presents the losses of plant material caused by the evaluation under conditions of the Czech Republic. Every year around 30–40% of the genotypes were harvested. These genotypes have demonstrated their viability in the conditions of the Czech Republic. In 2014, a new variety of *Sorghum bicolor* 'Ruzrok' bred for conditions in the Czech Republic was registered (**Appendix III**). Considerable interest of breeders (abroad) is enjoyed by sorghum hybrids with Sudan grass (*Sorghum bicolor* x *Sorghum sudanense*) where there might be considerable variability between varieties. In the conditions of the Czech Republic, this is probably the most common form that is usually used for the production of high-quality silage, haylage with high hemicellulose content, direct feeding, grazing cattle, and biogas production. The aim of intensive breeding in both sorghum species suitable for silage production is BMR form (brown midrib)—the form of cytoplasmic mutation (CMS). These varieties possess higher digestibility where the outward characteristic is brown midrib.

5. Uses of foxtail millet and sorghum

Foxtail millet is a multipurpose crop. It is suitable for human consumption (grain) and livestock nutrition (grain, forage). For human consumption, the grain must be dehulled in the mills because the kernel and palea knit together. Published studies reported higher nutritional value than rice [50]. Tables 4–9 show the evaluation of three foxtail millet genotypes in 2002–2003 cultivated in the conditions of the Czech Republic (CRI, Prague Ruzyně). The numbers are the average values from two successive years. The content of crude proteins (11.42%) was higher than in rice, wheat, or corn. The ratio of pure protein is up to 91.5% [51, 52]. From protein fractions, the albumins and globulins represented 13.1%, prolamins 39.4%, glutelins 9.9%. According to the gluten content, foxtail millet's grains are considered for a gluten-free diet [52]. The content and composition of amino acids is beneficial for human health, as most of the cereals have low lysine content [53]. The content of essential amino acids (threonine, valine, methionine, isoleucine, leucine, and phenylalanine) presented in foxtail millet grains is about 41% higher than rice, 65% higher than in wheat flour, and approximately 51.1% more than in corn. These amino acids are important for poultry nutrition. As stated by Pack et al. [54], lysine, methionine, threonine, and cysteine are essential for nutrition and affordable cost for the preparation of animal feed. This crop can contribute to a natural increase of these substances in animal feed. The observed content of fat ranged from 5.02 to 5.56%; similar results were published by Zhang et al. [55], which is more than it is known in wheat and maize. There is a higher content of unsaturated fatty acids (namely linoleic, linolenic, and gadoleic) compared with fatty acids of maize [56]. Carbohydrate content is 72.8% and it is lower than in rice, wheat, and maize. The size of starch granules ranges from 0.8 to 9.6 μm. The content of amylose and amylopectin depends on the variety. There are so-called waxy varieties with high content of amylopectin or with low or high content of amylose [57]. Zhu [58] observed millet as a starch supplying crop that appeared strategically promising. The content of minerals iron, zinc, copper, and magnesium is higher in comparison with rice and wheat. The observed content of vitamins was consistent with published results of Saleh et al. [59], whereas the content of

Ca is considered on a similar level as in rice and wheat. Seeds of foxtail millet are rich in Se and the fibre content (11%) is four times higher than that of rice.

		Dry matter	Ash	Fat	Protein	Fibre
Year	2002	93.83 ± 2.08a	3.23 ± 0.22a	5.20 ± 0.21a	12.67 ± 0.32a	18.83 ± 0.42a
	2003	93.27 ± 0.10a	2.96 ± 0.10a	5.30 ± 0.43a	12.07 ± 0.08a	15.91 ± 1.81a
Genotype	01Z230023	92.33 ± 1.17a	2.99 ± 0.01a	5.15 ± 0.13a	12.48 ± 0.46a	17.09 ± 2.28a
	01Z230002	94.41 ± 1.54a	3.19 ± 0.23a	5.56 ± 0.29a	12.45 ± 0.64a	18.60 ± 1.00a
	01Z230014	93.92 ± 0.82a	3.11 ± 0.36a	5.02 ± 0.06a	12.18 ± 0.18a	16.43 ± 2.93a

Table 4. Basic nutritional components (g 100 g^{-1} of sample) of foxtail millet grains (data evaluated in the Gene Bank, CRI, Prague Ruzyně).

		B1	B2	Niacin	Pantothenic acid	B6	Carotenoids
Year	2002	0.40 ± 0.01a	0.10 ± 0.01a	2.73 ± 0.06a	1.31 ± 0.19a	0.30 ± 0.03b	0.67 ± 0.08a
	2003	0.39 ± 0.04a	0.12 ± 0.00a	3.23 ± 0.15b	1.13 ± 0.10a	0.24 ± 0.02a	0.73 ± 0.06a
Genotype	01Z230023	0.39 ± 0.04a	0.10 ± 0.02a	2.95 ± 0.35a	1.13 ± 0.13a	0.25 ± 0.03a	0.78 ± 0.04b
	01Z230002	0.41 ± 0.03a	0.11 ± 0.01a	3.10 ± 0.42a	1.34 ± 0.28a	0.28 ± 0.06a	0.70 ± 0.03ab
	01Z230014	0.38 ± 0.01a	0.11 ± 0.02a	2.90 ± 0.28a	1.21 ± 0.02a	0.29 ± 0.04a	0.64 ± 0.06a

Table 5. Vitamin content (mg 100 g^{-1} of sample) in foxtail millet (data evaluated in the Gene Bank, CRI, Prague Ruzyně).

In comparison with other cereals (wheat and maize), the foxtail millet grains reached higher values of some evaluated nutritional components. According to Zhang and Liu [60], foxtail millet demonstrated remarkable peroxyl radical scavenging capacity and cellular antioxidative activity due to its content of phenolic compounds, phenolic acids, and carotenoids, and it is considered as a valuable cereal with potential in the prevention and management of cardiovascular and geriatric diseases, as well as cancers. Foxtail millet is considered as an ideal crop for producing food for diabetics.

		Aspartic acid	Threonine	Serine	Glutamic	Proline	Glycin
Year	2002	0.76 ± 0.07a	0.39 ± 0.02a	0.47 ± 0.03a	1.94 ± 0.12a	1.07 ± 0.15a	0.27 ± 0.03a
	2003	0.80 ± 0.01a	0.45 ± 0.02b	0.45 ± 0.03a	2.07 ± 0.05a	0.87 ± 0.17a	0.30 ± 0.01a
Genotype	01Z230023	0.75 ± 0.09a	0.40 ± 0.04a	0.46 ± 0.04a	1.96 ± 0.22a	0.99 ± 0.11a	0.26 ± 0.03a
	01Z230002	0.79 ± 0.00a	0.44 ± 0.05a	0.46 ± 0.04a	2.06 ± 0.04a	0.93 ± 0.27a	0.29 ± 0.03a
	01Z230014	0.81 ± 0.01a	0.42 ± 0.03a	0.46 ± 0.03a	2.00 ± 0.02a	1.00 ± 0.27a	0.30 ± 0.00a

Table 6. Amino acid content (g 100 g^{-1} of sample) in foxtail millet grains (data evaluated in the Gene Bank, CRI, Prague Ruzyně).

		Alanine	Valine	Methionine	Isoleucine	Leucine	Tyrosine	Phenyl-alanine
Year	2002	0.94 ± 0.08a	0.50 ± 0.02a	0.29 ± 0.04a	0.50 ± 0.10a	1.53 ± 0.15a	0.37 ± 0.05a	0.64 ± 0.05a
	2003	0.95 ± 0.03a	0.54 ± 0.03a	0.18 ± 0.06a	0.54 ± 0.10a	1.31 ± 0.10a	0.30 ± 0.02a	0.78 ± 0.03b
Genotype	01Z230023	0.92 ± 0.09a	0.51 ± 0.04a	0.22 ± 0.04a	0.53 ± 0.16a	1.32 ± 0.05a	0.32 ± 0.02a	0.67 ± 0.12a
	01Z230002	0.97 ± 0.01a	0.54 ± 0.05a	0.22 ± 0.15a	0.52 ± 0.12a	1.42 ± 0.28a	0.33 ± 0.02a	0.72 ± 0.07a
	01Z230014	0.96 ± 0.05a	0.51 ± 0.00a	0.27 ± 0.05a	0.51 ± 0.04a	1.52 ± 0.14a	0.36 ± 0.11a	0.74 ± 0.11a

Table 6. (continues).

		Histidine	Lysine	Arginine	Cysteine	Total
Year	2002	0.28 ± 0.02a	0.18 ± 0.02a	0.38 ± 0.03a	0.22 ± 0.00a	10.75 ± 0.90a
	2003	0.26 ± 0.09a	0.23 ± 0.01a	0.59 ± 0.02b	0.24 ± 0.04a	10.86 ± 0.47a
Genotype	01Z230023	0.31 ± 0.08a	0.19 ± 0.05a	0.48 ± 0.19a	0.24 ± 0.02a	10.53 ± 1.17a
	01Z230002	0.25 ± 0.06a	0.21 ± 0.03a	0.48 ± 0.14a	0.21 ± 0.02a	10.84 ± 0.58a
	01Z230014	0.24 ± 0.05a	0.21 ± 0.01a	0.49 ± 0.11a	0.24 ± 0.03a	11.04 ± 0.35a

Table 6. (continues).

		Myristic (14:0)	Palmitic (16:0)	Palmitooleic (16:1)	Stearic (18:0)	Oleic (18:1)	Linoleic (18:2)
Year	2002	0.13 ± 0.03b	7.99 ± 0.80a	0.13 ± 0.02a	1.26 ± 0.15a	16.31 ± 2.00a	69.77 ± 1.50a
	2003	0.09 ± 0.02a	9.47 ± 0.98a	0.14 ± 0.02a	1.40 ± 0.08a	15.59 ± 1.34a	69.67 ± 0.19a
Genotype	01Z230023	0.13 ± 0.04a	8.85 ± 2.21a	0.14 ± 0.01a	1.39 ± 0.06a	16.70 ± 2.70a	68.89 ± 1.12a
	01Z230002	0.09 ± 0.02a	8.14 ± 0.45a	0.15 ± 0.02a	1.33 ± 0.23a	16.25 ± 1.26a	70.23 ± 1.06a
	01Z230014	0.11 ± 0.03a	9.21 ± 0.49a	0.12 ± 0.00a	1.27 ± 0.13a	14.91 ± 0.08a	70.06 ± 0.28a

Table 7. Fatty acid content (g 100 g^{-1} of fatty acid) in the oil of foxtail millet grains (data evaluated in the Gene Bank, CRI, Prague Ruzyně).

		Linolenic (18:3)	Arachic (20:0)	Gadoleic (20:1)	Behenic (22:0)
Year	2002	3.04 ± 0.46a	0.46 ± 0.03a	0.39 ± 0.02a	0.36 ± 0.05a
	2003	2.59 ± 0.27a	0.41 ± 0.05a	0.36 ± 0.13a	0.24 ± 0.03a
Genotype	01Z230023	2.58 ± 0.09a	0.43 ± 0.09a	0.35 ± 0.06a	0.32 ± 0.13a
	01Z230002	2.81 ± 0.72a	0.43 ± 0.01a	0.32 ± 0.07a	0.27 ± 0.07a
	01Z230014	3.06 ± 0.33a	0.46 ± 0.01a	0.46 ± 0.07a	0.31 ± 0.05a

Table 7. (continues).

		Na	K	Ca	Mg	P
Year	2002	2.73 ± 0.85a	401.33 ± 29.54a	18.07 ± 1.40a	127.00 ± 3.46a	353.33 ± 10.02a
	2003	3.37 ± 0.85a	364.00 ± 7.21a	18.27 ± 1.66a	124.33 ± 5.86a	359.00 ± 16.82a
Genotype	01Z230023	3.95 ± 0.35b	368.50 ± 3.54a	17.50 ± 1.41a	125.50 ± 4.95a	364.50 ± 10.61a
	01Z230002	2.90 ± 0.71ab	379.50 ± 33.23a	17.85 ± 1.91a	127.00 ± 5.66a	353.50 ± 16.26a
	01Z230014	2.30 ± 0.28a	400.00 ± 42.43a	19.15 ± 0.92a	124.50 ± 6.36a	350.50 ± 14.85a

Table 8. Content of mineral components (mg 100 g^{-1} of sample) in foxtail millet grains (data evaluated in the Gene Bank, CRI, Prague Ruzyně).

		Zn	Fe	Cu	Mn
Year	2002	3.80 ± 0.10a	6.73 ± 1.86a	0.54 ± 0.04a	1.37 ± 0.15a
	2003	4.10 ± 0.10b	3.30 ± 0.26a	0.63 ± 0.09a	1.30 ± 0.17a
Genotype	01Z230023	3.90 ± 0.28a	4.65 ± 2.19a	0.55 ± 0.06a	1.30 ± 0.14a
	01Z230002	4.05 ± 0.21a	6.00 ± 3.96a	0.66 ± 0.11a	1.50 ± 0.00a
	01Z230014	3.90 ± 0.14a	4.40 ± 1.13a	0.55 ± 0.02a	1.20 ± 0.00a

Table 8. (continues).

Foxtail millet can also be used as an animal feed. Tables 9 and 10 show basic nutritional composition and amino acid composition of foxtail green biomass. The straw is ideal for cattle because of its high nutritional value (the protein content of 6.0%, 26.0% simple sugars; xylogen 24.2%; 42.2% fibrin), which is much higher than in many other crops. Moreover, foxtail millet straw is relatively soft and easily digestible for cattle [51].

ECN	Dry matter (%)	Ash (%)	Organic matter (%)	Fibre (%)	N × 6.25	N × 5.93	Fat (%)	Nitrogen-free substances (%)
01Z2300003	100	2.95	97.05	9.97	14.3	13.31	4.25	68.8
01Z2300009	100	2.23	97.77	8.7	16.66	15.8	4.2	68.21
01Z2300010	100	3.38	96.62	8.95	15.76	14.96	4.49	67.41

Table 9. Basic nutritional components in green biomass of foxtail millet grains (data evaluated in the Gene Bank, CRI, Prague Ruzyně).

	g kg^{-1} of original value														
ECN	asp	thr	ser	glu	pro	gly	ala	val	ile	leu	tyr	phe	his	lys	arg
01Z2300003	2.1	0.79	1.4	5.2	2.42	0.73	2.49	1.32	1.14	3.92	0.68	1.42	0.83	0.58	0.88
01Z2300009	2.63	4.7	1.39	6.15	3.5	0.93	3.6	1.4	1.44	4.79	0.89	1.81	1.4	0.72	1.27
01Z2300010	1.71	0.65	0.99	4.57	2.23	0.69	2.16	1.41	1.2	3.37	0.66	1.26	0.75	0.48	0.66

Table 10. Amino acid content in green biomass of foxtail millet grains (data evaluated in the Gene Bank, CRI, Prague Ruzyně).

Possibilities for sorghum utilisation are very broad. In the food industry, it is used for the production of sorghum sugar syrups, sweets, ethanol, alcoholic beverages, and beer because of easy and quick fermentation. The preparation of purée from flour and groats in combination with meat and vegetables is widespread [61]. Industrial use of sorghum flour is for the production of adhesives, oils, and starch [62]. Recently, a high increase in the production of ethanol as a fuel from biomass was recorded [63]. Sorghum is also suitable as a high-quality forage crop because of its high sugar content, very good digestibility, and high yields of green silage. Manifold technical sorghum is the raw material for the production of brushes and brooms.

Variety	Content of crude protein	Fat	BNLV	Fibre	Ash
Grain	12.8	3.3	76	5.9	2
Sugar	14.2	3.7	73.6	6	2.6
Technical	13.7	3.6	73	7.5	2.2

Table 11. Chemical composition of sorghum grains (%) from the collection of genetic resources in the Gene Bank, CRI Prague Ruzyně (2011).

The content of nutritional components differs depending on the cultivation site and conditions. **Table 11** shows original data as a result of chemical composition analysis of cultivated sorghum varieties in the Gene Bank (CRI, Prague Ruzyně). The content of starch is similar to maize at around 70%, protein content 8–16%, fat content 3.3%, minerals 1.9%, and crude fibre 1.9% [64]. As is commonly known, the content of proteins is strongly affected by nitrogen fertilisation; it elevates the content of prolamin fraction, which is known as karirin in the case of sorghum. This fraction is poor in lysine, arginine, histidin, and tryptophan and rich in prolin and glutamin. Rajki-Siklósi [49] presented a protein content in sorghum seeds from 10.0 to 10.7%. The tannin (proanthocyanidin) content together with some of the others is considered as a negative component, which negatively influenced digestibility. The amino acid composition of sorghum seeds is variable, according to published studies [65–67], depending on genotypes and cultivation localities. Lysine in commonly available genotypes covers almost 40% of the recommended dose of this essential amino acid, especially for children in developing countries. High lysine genotypes have higher content of lysine and the total content of amino acids is nutritionally more beneficial [68]. Interest in the cultivation of sorghum in Central Europe is growing with respect to climate change, utilisation for feeding purposes, and in human nutrition for the possibility of its use in gluten-free diets. There are genotypic differences when grain sorghum varieties compared to sugar sorghum show a favourable composition of protein fractions, a higher proportion of nutritionally valuable albumin and globulins, and a lower content of prolamins. Results of Petr et al. [52] confirmed the suitability of sorghum for a gluten-free diet.

Among the biologically active substances in sorghum is the prized content of phenolic acids, which are represented as protocatechuic acid, hydroxybenzoic, vanillic, caffeic, ferulic, and cinnamon. These acids are important for their high antioxidant properties. From the minerals in sorghum, there are interesting contents of phosphorus, magnesium, iron, zinc, copper, manganese, molybdenum, and chromium. Sorghum further comprises vitamins B1, B6, beta carotene, folacin, and pantothenic acid, which is important for metabolic processing of nutrients and irreplaceable for hormone synthesis [69]. The possibility of higher use for food purposes exist in Europe, which is at a low level at the moment.

In the Czech Republic, varieties and hybrids of sorghum are primarily used for feed and biogas production [70]. Traditional varieties of sorghum are now being replaced by new hybrids with favourable agrotechnical and nutritional properties. In recent years, the hybrids most used for these purposes are derived from crosses of grain or sugar sorghum with Sudan grass. Their advantage is the high-quality production of green matter. Intensive breeding has managed to dismantle the previously high content of alkaloid durin and increase the digestibility of organic nutrients.

In 2009 and 2010, field experiments with selected sorghum materials were carried out at the Gene Bank (CRI, Prague Ruzyně). The size of the field was 4.5 m^2 in three repetitions. The plant materials used were commercial varieties of sorghum provided by the companies Seed Service, Saatbau Linz, and Syngenta. Some of the tested materials were obtained from the Gene Bank (CRI, Prague Ruzyně). The results of the experiments are summarised in Tables 12 and 13.

Variety	Height	Biomass	Content of essential nutrition in % dry matter (d.m.)				
	(cm)	(kg m $^{-2}$)	N	P	K	Ca	Mg
Čirok	200.53 ± 27.43	7.69 ± 2.46	1.86 ± 0.42	0.25 ± 0.07	3.25 ± 1.13	0.71 ± 0.11	0.24 ± 0.04
Goliath [1]	228.67 ± 22.27	10.10 ± 0.93	1.82 ± 0.40	0.25 ± 0.08	3.41 ± 1.24	0.70 ± 0.09	0.25 ± 0.02
Sucrosorgo 506 [2]	209.50 ± 24.34	8.62 ± 2.16	1.87 ± 0.29	0.26 ± 0.07	3.40 ± 0.97	0.69 ± 0.12	0.24 ± 0.03
Nutri Honey [3]	199.33 ± 20.85	7.18 ± 1.37	1.75 ± 0.37	0.23 ± 0.05	2.58 ± 0.71	0.65 ± 0.11	0.23 ± 0.03
Latte [4]	197.67 ± 25.01	7.96 ± 3.60	1.70 ± 0.55	0.25 ± 0.06	2.92 ± 1.09	0.63 ± 0.09	0.22 ± 0.04
Honey Graze BMR [5]	194.83 ± 14.80	5.60 ± 1.46	1.83 ± 0.53	0.23 ± 0.08	3.52 ± 1.79	0.76 ± 0.05	0.24 ± 0.04
Big Kahuna BMR [6]	173.17 ± 30.04	6.71 ± 2.25	2.17 ± 0.37	0.29 ± 0.08	3.66 ± 0.73	0.82 ± 0.06	0.28 ± 0.02

1. Goliath—early hybrid, suitable for biogas production.
2. Sucrosorgo 506—hybrid, high yields of green biomass even in places not suitable for corn silage.
3. Nutri Honey—hybrid of sorghum and Sudan grass, suitable for forage and grazing.
4. Latte—forage variety, high resistance to drought.
5. Honey Graze BMR—hybrid suitable for making silage, hay, green feed or grazing; a lower lignin content.
6. Big Kahuna BMR—hybrid for silage, photosensitive to short-day.

Table 12. Evaluated parameters of biomass in sorghum varieties; mean values from 2009 to 2010.

Variety	Height	Biomass	Content of essential nutrients in % dry matter (d.m.)				
	(cm)	(kg m^{-2})	N	P	K	Ca	Mg
K−81	291.00 ± 4.58a	26.08 ± 1.97a	1.00 ± 0.04abc	0.15 ± 0.01ab	1.03 ± 0.06abc	0.47 ± 0.01c	0.21 ± 0.01a
Kecskemeti	314.67 ± 4.51a	26.24 ± 5.84a	0.97 ± 0.10bc	0.15 ± 0.01ab	0.86 ± 0.07b	0.45 ± 0.02bc	0.22 ± 0.02a
SO−29	302.33 ± 7.02a	26.61 ± 2.74a	1.16 ± 0.10abc	0.19 ± 0.02a	1.08 ± 0.05a	0.36 ± 0.02a	0.17 ± 0.00a
GK 4 Zsofia	308.67 ± 7.57a	24.07 ± 4.41a	1.22 ± 0.09ab	0.18 ± 0.02ab	0.89 ± 0.03bc	0.43 ± 0.02abc	0.20 ± 0.02a
6−without tannin (sugar)	304.00 ± 19.70a	20.04 ± 3.39a	1.26 ± 0.12a	0.18 ± 0.04ab	1.09 ± 0.07a	0.40 ± 0.03abc	0.19 ± 0.03a
21/00	308.00 ± 14.00a	29.51 ± 7.21a	1.25 ± 0.15ab	0.20 ± 0.04a	0.89 ± 0.12bc	0.39 ± 0.04ab	0.19 ± 0.03a
56/01	317.00 ± 7.00a	28.25 ± 4.51a	1.17 ± 0.08abc	0.17 ± 0.01ab	1.04 ± 0.15ac	0.43 ± 0.05abc	0.18 ± 0.03a
GK 5 Zsofia	294.67 ± 12.66a	20.25 ± 1.83a	1.27 ± 0.06a	0.18 ± 0.01ab	1.10 ± 0.08a	0.39 ± 0.04ab	0.19 ± 0.01a
Latte	312.67 ± 9.07a	28.51 ± 3.51a	0.89 ± 0.05c	0.12 ± 0.00b	1.16 ± 0.09a	0.37 ± 0.02a	0.18 ± 0.01a

Values with different letter indexes were statistically significantly different $P \leq 0.05$.

Table 13. Evaluated parameters of biomass in sorghum varieties; mean values from 2009–2010.

When the green biomass is mowed from the beginning of flowering, the protein content of the forage is very high, comparable with the content of the other young grasses or alfalfa. In that growth phase, the plants have a high content of soluble fibre, which decreases progressively with aging of the plants and the protein content is diluted as well. Significant lignification occurs after flowering of the plants.

Sorghums generally ensure high yields of biomass in appropriate conditions. The harvest depends on the purposes of cultivation. Achieved yields of sorghum biomass in field experiments performed by the CRI and analysis of other outcome measures are summarised in Tables 14 and 15.

Locality/variety	Sudanense grass	Hyso*	Grain sorghum	Sugar sorghum
Ruzyně	9.4	11.9	12.4	8.7
Troubsko	26.7	27.2	31.2	9.3
Lukavec	–	–	21.9	3.3
Chomutov	–	12.8	5.3	7.4
Mean	18.0	17.3	17.7	7.2

*variety hybrid between Sudanense grass and technical sorghum

Table 14. Average yields of biomass dry matter (t. ha^{-1}) in tested sorghum genotypes in the period 1993–2004.

The experiments obtained average yields of dry matter of biomass from 27.06 t ha^{-1} in Troubsko to 5.14 t ha^{-1} in Lukavec. In Lukavec, there were not suitable conditions for tested sorghum hybrids. Without consideration of these results, the average yield of dry matter of biomass in all genotypes was 15.56 t ha^{-1} (data not shown). The presented average yield of dry matter of biomass was influenced by values obtained from sugar sorghum genotypes, which were low in all the tested localities (**Table 14**). From the tested sorghum genotypes all reached similar yields on average (18.02 t ha^{-1} Sudan grass, 17.71 t ha^{-1} grain sorghum and 17.29 t ha^{-1} "Hyso"). In the comparison of localities, the highest yields of biomass were gained in all tested genotypes in the warmest locality in Troubsko and, in contrast, the lowest yields were obtained in Lukavec, the coldest locality. Sorghum positively reacted to graded doses of nitrogen fertilisation. In our tests, the yield of biomass was increased by around 13.3% in experimental plots fertilised with 60 kg ha^{-1} of N and around 17.0% in plots fertilised with 120 kg ha^{-1} of N in comparison with un-fertilised plots. Similarly, experiments in Germany confirmed high yields of sorghum from 15 to 20 t ha^{-1} in warm localities with a sum of temperatures higher than 2000°C. Also, the sowing rate had a significant effect on biomass yield (data not shown). In all localities, higher yield was obtained by the application of a sowing rate of 60 seeds per m^2.

The influence of locality and nitrogen fertilisation on yields on above ground biomass was evaluated. The effect of the harvest time on water content in the harvested plant material, the loss of biomass over the winter period, the content of essential nutrients and energy content in plants were all observed. Also, the comparison of the monitored genotypes (varieties) of sorghum in terms of suitability for burning and the impact of the date of harvest on yield, water content, mineral content, and content in biomass were evaluated.

From the point of view of energy utilisation and storage of biomass, the content of the dry matter is important at harvest time. In an autumn harvest, the water content is high (around 66%). By postponing the harvest to spring time, the water content in plants is reduced but, due to plant morphology and high weight of panicles, lodging occurs resulting in losses of biomass.

The content of minerals in plants is one of the most important factors for the determination of nutrient uptake by yields, in terms of combustion of the biomass, the formation of biogas, etc. Generally, it can be said that the content of nitrogen in plants decreases with the age of the plants and the harvest time. In general, delaying harvest time also reduces the content of the monitored elements in the biomass.

In Europe (notably Germany, Austria, and Italy) where bioenergy is focused on biogas rather than ethanol, sorghum has recently drawn attention as a novel bioenergy crop. Maize is currently used in the Czech Republic for producing biogas. With respect to conserving and increasing the biodiversity of cultivated agriculture crops and eliminating the negative effects on the environment of monoculture cultivation of maize, the alternative crops are sought-after. Sorghum should be one suitable possibility. Sorghum is considered as a dry tolerant crop suitable for cultivation on light soils and arid areas [71]. Habyarinama et al. [72] proposed the development of drought tolerant sorghum hybrids in order to increase and stabilise biomass production in the Mediterranean region. Recently, Windpassinger et al. [73] stated that sorghum provided high yields of biomass suitable for silage production under temperate conditions. The interest in sorghum cultivation may increase in the future due to changing climate conditions in Central Europe.

Our experimental data of chemical composition and fermentations processes of the broad sorghum collection corresponded to [74–76]. The results obtained showed high variability in the chemical composition, and biogas production in different varieties and hybrids. This fact highlighted the importance of careful selection of suitable varieties and genotypes based on testing the sorghum collection at the Gene Bank of the CRI, Prague Ruzyně. **Table 15** presents comparative data of the evaluated sorghum and maize. Sorghums contained a high content of ash (approx. 50%), fibre (approx. 60%), lignin (approx. 30%), and a low content of protein (approx. 8%) and fat (approx. 30%). This is the reason for lower yields of methane and biogas from sorghum (mainly from hybrids) in comparison with maize (6–16%). However, from 1 ha of sorghum, it is possible to obtain a similar or even higher amount of biogas (mainly methane) thanks to the higher yields of dry matter of biomass. For these purposes, the selection of suitable genotypes is essential with the emphasis on early maturation for conditions in the Czech Republic.

Parameter	Sorghum	Maize
Ash (% in d.m.)	6–12	4–8
Crude protein (% in d.m.)	5–9	6–9
Carbohydrates total (% in d.m.)	8–18	8–18
Crude fat (% in d.m.)	1–3	2–4
Crude fibre (% in d.m.)	32–44	20–28
Neutral detergent fibre (NDF) (% in d.m.)	48–62	32–44
Hemicelluloses (% in d.m.)	12–18	12–16
Lignin (% in d.m.)	3–6	2–5
Losses of dry matter in silage (% in d.m.)	2–8	2–6
Yield of biogas ($Nm^3.t^{-1}$ of d.m.)	420–620	400–710
Methane concentration (%)	52–55	52–55
Methane yield (Nm^3 t^{-1} in d.m.)	220–340	210–390
Methane yield (Nm^3 t^{-1} of org. d m.)	240–380	230–440
Average yields of dry matter of biomass (t ha^{-1})	9–22	8–18
Methane yields (Nm^3 ha^{-1})	2000–7500	1700–7000

Table 15. Mean values of sorghum biomass composition, biogas, and biomass in comparison with maize.

Field experiments in four localities (Ruzyně, Lukavec, Chomutov, and Troubsko) in the years from 1993 to 2004 with selected sorghum genotypes (Sudan grass, "Hyso," grain sorghum, and sugar sorghum) considered for potential energy are shown in **Table 16**; they were conducted under three different nitrogen doses (0, 60, 120 kg ha^{-1}) and one or two levels of seed rates (40 and 60 germinating seeds per 1 m^2) by spacing 25 cm and two harvests period in the autumn and spring.

Locality/variant	Ruzyně	Troubsko	Lukavec	Chomutov	Mean
Average N0	10.5	26.1	2.3	10.0	12.2
Average N1	11.7	27.2	6.1	11.5	14.1
Average N2	12.2	27.9	7.0	11.8	14.7
Average V1	10.9	27.0	4.4	12.2	13.6
Average V2	12.0	27.2	5.9	10.1	13.8
Mean	11.5	27.1	5.1	11.1	13.7

Notes: Mineral nitrogen fertilization: N0 = 0, N1 = 60, N2 = 120 kg ha^1.
Supposed no. of plants per m^2: V1 = 40, V2 = 60.

Table 16. Average yields of dry matter of biomass (t ha^{-1}) according to variants in experimental fields in the period 1993–2004.

6. Conclusion

Foxtail millet has a long history of cultivation around the world and is valued for its nutritional content and health promoting properties, its ability to grow under low-input conditions, and its tolerance to extreme environmental stresses. Similarly, sorghum has recently attracted attention as a novel bioenergy crop. In a world facing limited natural resources and climate change, we considered both mentioned species as having great potential for food use in the case of foxtail millet and for biomass production in case of sorghum in arid and semi-arid areas of the Czech Republic and further for other areas of Central European countries. Genetic resources of both species can provide genotypic and phenotypic variability for conservation and exploitation of biodiversity in the context of warmer weather affecting global agricultural production.

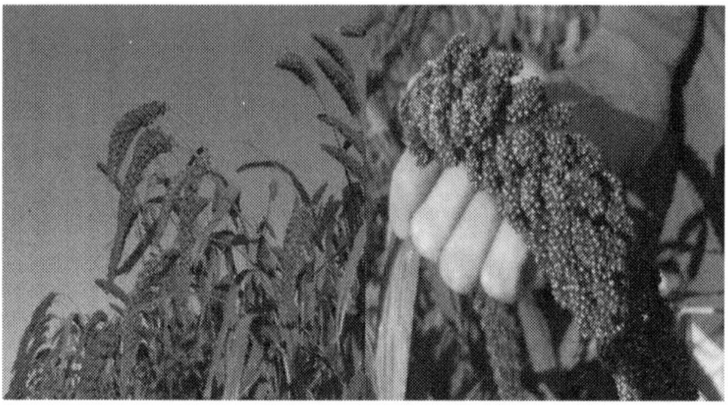

Appendix I. New variety of *Setaria italica* 'Ruberit' bred for conditions of the Central Europe.

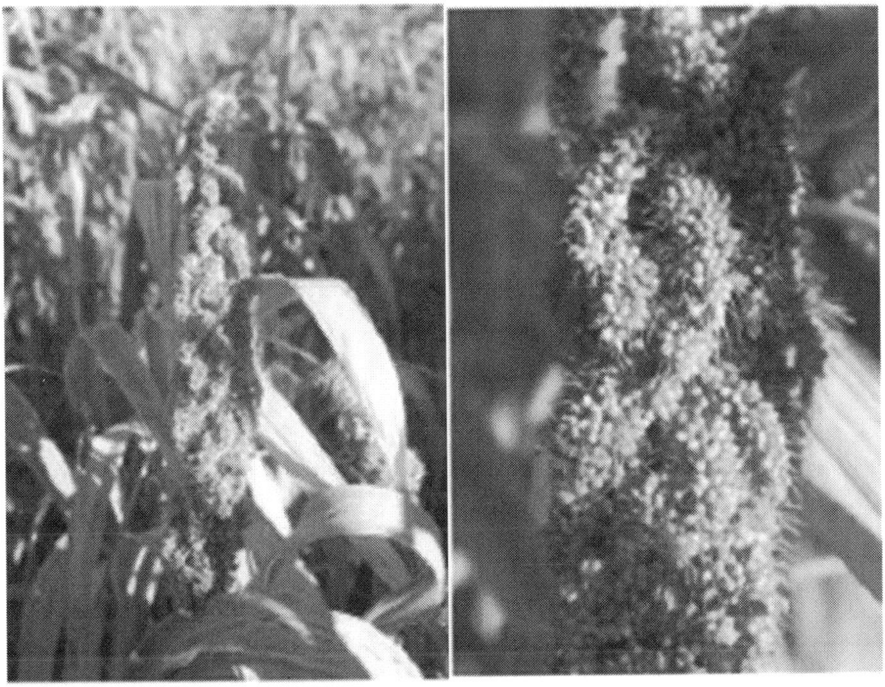

Appendix II. New genotype of *Setaria italica* 'Rucereus' bred for conditions of the Central Europe.

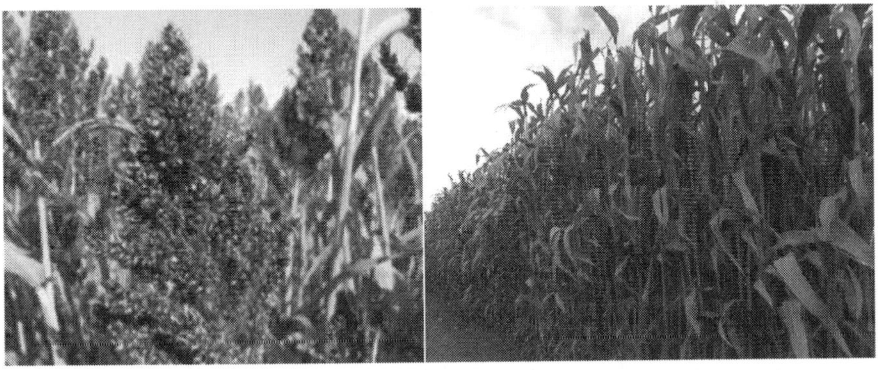

Appendix III. New variety of *Sorghum bicolor* 'Ruzrok' bred for conditions of the Central Europe.

Acknowledgements

This work was finantially supported by National Programme on Conservation and Utilization of Plant, Animal and Microbial Genetic resources (Projects no. 206553/2011-MZE-17253) and the Ministry of Agriculture of the Czech Republic (Projects no. RO0415).

Author details

Jiří Hermuth[1], Dagmar Janovská[1], Petra Hlásná Čepková[1], Sergej Usťak[2], Zdeněk Strašil[2] and Zdislava Dvořáková[3]

1 Crop Research Institute, Gene Bank, Drnovská 507, Prague 6 Ruzyně, Czech Republic

2 Crop Research Institute, Technologies for Sustainable Agriculture and Landscape Restoration, Drnovská 507, Prague 6 Ruzyně, Czech Republic

3 Czech University of Life Sciences Prague, Faculty of Tropical AgriSciences, Kamýcká 129, Prague 6, Suchdol, Czech Republic

References

[1] Belton, P. S.; Taylor, J. R. N. Sorghum and millets: protein sources for Africa. Trends in Food Science & Technology. 2003;15(2):94–98. DOI: 10.1016/j.tifs.2003.09.002

[2] McKevith, B. Nutrional aspects of cereals. British Nutrition Foundation Nutrition Bulletin. 2004;29:111–142.

[3] FAOSTAT. Statistical database of the Food and Agricultural Organization of the United Nations [Internet]. 2005. Available from: http://faostat.fao.org [Accessed: 2012-04-19].

[4] Winch, T. Growing Food. A Guide to Food Production. 1st ed. Netherlands: Springer; 2006. 333 p. DOI: 10.1007/978-1-4020-4975-0

[5] Matz, S. A. Other cereal grains. In: Matz, S. A., editors. The Chemistry and Technology of Cereals as Food and Feed. 2nd ed. Westport: The AVI Publishing Company; 1991. p. 259–284.

[6] Lasztity, R. Millet proteins. In: Lasztity, R., editors. The Chemistry of Cereal Proteins. 2nd ed. USA: CRC Press; 1996. p. 295–308.

[7] Obilana, A. B., Manyasa, E. Millets. In: Belton, P. S.; Taylor, J. R. N., editors. Pseudo-cereals and Less Common Cereals: Grain Properties and Utilization Potential. Heidelberg: Springer; 2002. p. 127–130.

[8] Taylor, J. R. N.; Schober, T. J.; Bean, S. R. Review. Novel food and non-food uses for sorghum and millets. Journal of Cereal Science. 2006;44:252–271. DOI: 10.1016/j.jcs.2006.06.009

[9] National Research Council. Lost Crops of Africa. Vol. 1. Grains. Washington, DC: National Academy Press; 1996.

[10] Li, Y.; Wu, S. Z. Traditional maintenance and multiplication of foxtail millet (*Setaria italica* (L.) P. Beauv.) landraces in China. Euphytica. 1996;87(1):33–38. DOI: 10.1007/BF00022961

[11] Brink, M., Belay, G. Plant Resources of Tropical Africa 1. Cereals and Pulses. Wageningen, Netherlands: PROTA Foundation; 2006. 298 p.

[12] Sakamoto, S. Origin and dispersal of common millet and foxtail millet. Japan Agricultural Research Quarterly. 1987;21:84–89.

[13] de Wet, J. M. J. *Eleusine coracana* (L.) Gaertn. In: Brink, M., Belay, G., editors. PROTA (Plant Resources of Tropical Africa/ Ressources végétales de l'Afrique tropicale). Wageningen [Internet]; 2006. Available from: http://database.prota.org/search.htm [Accessed 2012-03-19].

[14] Fukunaga, K.; Ichitani, K.; Kawase, M. Phylogenetic analysis of the rDNA intergenic spacer subrepeats and its implication for the domestication history of foxtail millet, *Setaria italica*. Theoretical and Applied Genetics. 2006;113(2):261–269. DOI: 10.1007/s00122-006-0291-5

[15] Rahayu, M.; Jansen, P. C. M. *Setaria italica* (L.) P. Beauvois cv. group foxtail millet. In: Grubben, G. J. H.; Partohardjono, S., editors. Plant Resources of South-East Asia No 10. Cereals. Leiden, The Netherlands: Backhuya Publishers; 1996. p. 127–130.

[16] Léder, I. Sorghum and millets. In: Füleky, G., editors. Cultivated Plants, Primarily as Food Sources, Encyclopedia of Life Support Systems (EOLSS) [online]. Developed under the Auspices of the UNESCO. Oxford, UK: Eolss Publishers; 2004. Available from: http://www.eolss.net [Accessed 2012-03-25].

[17] Ang, C. Y. W.; Liu, K.; Huang, Y.-W. Asian Foods: Science and Technology. New York: CRC Press; 1999. 546 p.

[18] Stenhouse, J. W.; Tippayaruk, J. L. *Sorghum bicolour* (L.) Moench. In: Grubben, G. J. H.; Partohardjono, S., editors. Plant Resources of South-East Asia No 10. Cereals. Leiden, Netherlands: Backhuys Publishers; 1996. p. 130–136.

[19] Doggett, H. Sorghum. 2nd ed. New York: John Wiley & Sons; 1988. 512 p.

[20] Balole, T. V.; Legwaila, G. M.; Brink, M.; Belay, G., editors. Plant Resources of Tropical Africa 1. Cereals and Pulses. Wageningen, Netherlands: Backhuys Publishers; 2006. p. 165–175.

[21] Baker, R. D. Millet Production. Guide A-414. New Mexico State University [Internet]; 2003. Available from: http://www.hort.purdue.edu/newcrop/nexus/setaria_italica_nex.html [Accessed 2012-04-12].

[22] Oelke, E. A.; Oplinger, E. S.; Putnam, D. H.; Durman, B. R.; Doll, J. D.; Undersander, D. J. Millets. In: Alternative Field Crops Manual [Internet]; 1990. Available from: www.hort.purdue.edu/newcrop/afcm/millet.html [Accessed 2015-09-29].

[23] Jayaraman, A.; Planik, S.; Rai, N. K.; Vidapu, S.; Sahu, P. P.; Lata, C.; Prasad, M. cDNA-AFLP Analysis reveals differential gene expression in response to salt stress in foxtail millet (*Setaria italica* L.). Molecular Biotechnology. 2008;40(3):241–251. DOI: 10.1007/s12033-008-9081-4

[24] Dekker, J. The foxtail (Setaria) species-group. Weed Science. 2003;51(5):641–656. DOI: 10.16.14/P2002-IR

[25] Duke, J. A. Sorghum bicolour (L.) Moench. In: Duke, J. A., editor. Handbook of Energy Crops [Internet]; 1983. Available from: http://www.hort.purdue.edu/newcrop/duke_energy/Sorghum_bicolour.html#Description [Accessed 2012-04-19].

[26] Duke, J. A. Handbook of Energy Crops [Internet]; 1983. Available from: http://www.hort.purdue.edu/newcrop/duke_energy/Echinochloa_crusgalli.html [Accessed 2012-04-13].

[27] Elzebroek, A. T. G.; Wind, K. Starch crops. In: Elzebroek, A. T. G.; Wind, K., editors. Guide to Cultivated Plants. Wallingford, UK: CABI; 2008. p. 316–397.

[28] Kimber, C. T. Origins of domesticated sorghum and its early diffusion to India and China. In: Smith, C. W.; Frederiksen, R. A., editors. Sorghum: Origin, History, Technology, and Production. USA: John Wiley & Sons, Inc.; 2000. p. 3–98.

[29] Reichert, R. D.; Nwasaru, M. A.; Mukuru, S. Z. Characterization of coloured grain sorghum lines and identification of high tannin lines with good dehulling characteristics. Cereal Chemistry. 1988;65(3):165–170.

[30] Rooney, L. W.; Serna-Seldivar, S. O. Sorghum. In: Kulp, K.; Ponte, J., editors. Handbook of Cereal Science and Technology. 2nd ed. New York: Marcel Dekker; 2007. p. 149–175.

[31] Wang, Z. M.; Devos, K. M.; Liu, C. J.; Wang, R. Q.; Gale, M. D. Construction of RFLP-based maps of foxtail millet, *Setaria italica* (L.) P. Beauv. Theoretical and Applied Genetics. 1998;96(1):31–36. DOI: 10.1007/s001220050705

[32] Upadhyaya, H. D.; Ramesh, S.; Sharma, S.; Singh, S. K.; Varshney, S. K.; Sarma, N. D. R. K.; Ravishankar, C. R.; Narasimhudu, Y.; Reddy, V. G.; Sahrawatt, K. L.; Dhanalakshmi, T. N.; Mgonja, M. A.; Parzies, H. K.; Gowda, C. L. L.; Singh, S. Genetic diversity for grain nutrients contents in a core collection of finger millet (*Eleusine coracana* (L.) Gaertn.) germplasm. Field Crops Research. 2011;121(1):42–52. DOI: 10.1016/j.fcr.2010.11.017

[33] Tian, B.; Wang, J.; Zhang, L.; Li, Y.; Wang, S.; Li, H. Assessment of resistance to lodging of landrace and improved cultivars in foxtail millet. Euphytica. 2010;172(3):295–302. DOI: 10.1007/s10681-009-9999-z

[34] Veeranagamallaiah, G.; Jyothsnakumari, G.; Thippeswamy, M.; Reddy, P. C. O.; Surabhi, G. K.; Sriranganayakulu, G.; Mahesh, Y.; Rajasekhar, B.; Madhurarekha, C.; Sudhakar, C. Proteomic analysis of salt stress responses in foxtail millet (*Setaria italica* L. cv. Prasad) seedlings. Plant Science. 2008;175(5):631–641. DOI: 10.1016/j.plantsci.2008.06.017

[35] Reddy, B. V. S.; Dakheel, A. J.; Ramesh, S.; Vadez, V.; Ibrahim, M.; Hebbar, M. Conventional Breeding Sorghum for Soil Salinity-Stress Tolerance. Documentation. Patancheru: International Crops Research Institute for the Semi-Arid Tropics; 2006.

[36] Rooney, L. W.; Serna-Seldivar, S. O. Sorghum. In: Kulp, K.; Ponte, J., editors. Handbook of Cereal Science and Technology. 2nd ed. New York: Marcel Dekker; 2007. p. 149–175.

[37] Makanda, I.; Tongoona, P.; Derera, J.; Sibiya, J.; Fato, P. Combining ability and cultivar superiority of sorghum germplasm for grain yield across tropical low- and mid-altitude environments. Field Crops Research. 2010;116(1–2):75–85. DOI: 10.1016/j.fcr.2009.11.015

[38] Haussmann, B. I. G.; Hess, D. E.; Welz, H. G.; Geiger, H. H. Improved methodologies for breeding striga-resistant sorghums. Field Crops Research. 2000;66(3):195–211. DOI: 10.1016/S0378-4290(00)00076-9

[39] Lawlor, D. W.; Cornic, G. Photosynthetic carbon assimilation and associated metabolism in relation to water deficits in higher plants. Plant, Cell and Environment. 2002;25(2):275–294. DOI: 10.1046/j.0016-8025.2001.00814.x

[40] Borrell, A. K.; Hammer, G. L.; Henzell, R. G. Does maintaining green leaf area in sorghum improve yield under drought? II. Dry matter production and yield. Crop Science. 2000;40(4):1037–1048.

[41] Harris, K.; Subudhi, P. K.; Borrell, A. K.; Jordan, D.; Rosenow, D.; Nguyen, H.; Klein, P.; Klein, R.; Mullet, J. Sorghum stay-green QTL individually reduce post-flowering drought-induced leaf senescence. Journal of Experimental Botany. 2007;58(2):327–338. DOI: 10.1093/jxb/erl225

[42] Cisneros López, E.; Mendpza-Onofre, L.; Mora-Aguilera, G.; Córdova-Téllez, L.; Livera-Muñoz, M. Cold tolerant sorghum hybrids and perental lines. III: Quality of seeds harvested from plants infected with *Fusarium verticillioides* (Sacc.) Nirenberg. Agrociencia. 2007;41:405–415.

[43] Kumar Swami, A.; Alam, S. I.; Sengupta, N.; Sarin, R. Differential proteomic analysis of salt stress response in Sorghum bicolor leaves. Environmental and Experimental Botany. 2011;71(2):321–328. DOI: 10.1016/j.envexpbot.2010.12.017

[44] Yang, X.; Zhang, J.; Perry, L.; Ma, Z.; Wan, Z.; Li, M.; Diao, X.; Lu, H. From the modern to the archaeological: starch grains from millets and their wild relatives in China. Journal of Archaeological Science. 2012;39(2):247–254. DOI: 10.1016/j.jas.2011.09.001

[45] Ambekar, S. S.; Kamatar, M. Y.; Ganesamurthy, K.; Ghorade, R. B.; Saxena, U.; Chand, P.; Jadav, B. D.; Das, I. K.; Nageshwararao, T. G.; Audilakshmi, S.; Seetharama, N. Genetic enhancement of Sorghum (*Sorghum bicolor* (L) Moench) for grain mould resistance: II. Breeding for grain mould resistance. Crop Protection. 2011;30(7):759–764. DOI: 10.1016/j.cropro.2010.06.024

[46] Audilakshmi, L.; Das, I. K.; Ghorade, R. B.; Mane, P. N.; Kamatar, M. Y.; Narayana, Y. D.; Seetharama, N. Genetic improvement of sorghum for grain mould resistance: I. Performance of sorghum recombinant inbred lines for grain mould reactions across environments. Crop Protection. 2011;30(7):735–758. DOI: 10.1016/j.cropro.2010.12.024

[47] Pande, S.; Thakur, R. P.; Karunakar, R. I.; Bandyopadhyay, R.; Reddy, B. V. S. Development of screening methods and identification of stable resistance to anthracnose in sorghum. Field Crop Research. 1994;38(3):157–166. DOI: 10.1016/0378-4290(94)90087-6

[48] Girijashankar, V.; Sharma, H. C.; Sharma, K. K.; Swathisree, V.; Prasad, L. S.; Bhat, B. V.; Royer, M.; Secundo, B. C.; Narasu, M. L.; Altosaar, I.; Seetharama, N. Development of transgenic sorghum for insect resistance against the spotted stem borer (*Chilo partellus*). Plant Cell Reports. 2005;24(9):513–522. DOI: 10.1007/s00299-005-0947-7

[49] Rajki-Siklosi, E. Examination of sorghum fibre and sugar content in Hungary. In: European Seminar on Perspectives of Sorghum in Europe. Sorghum for Energy and Industry; Toulouse, France; 1996. p. 49–55.

[50] Verma, S., Srivastava, S., Tiwari, N. Comparative study on nutritional and sensory quality of barnyard and foxtail millet food products with traditional rice products. Journal of Food Science and Technology. 2015;52(8):5147–5155. DOI: 10.1007/s13197-014-1617-y

[51] AU: Please provide publisher location for Ref. [51].Cheng, R.; Dong Z. Cereals in China. In: He, Z.; Bonjean, P. A., editors. Breeding and Production of Foxtail Millet in China. CIMMYT; 2010. p. 87–95.

[52] Petr, J.; Michalík, I.; Tláskalová-Hogenová, H.; Capouchová, I.; Faměra, O.; Urminská, D.; Tučková, L.; Knoblochová, H. Extension of the spektra of plant products for the diet in coeliac disease. Czech Journal of Food Science. 2003;21(2):8–15.

[53] Amadou, I.; Gounga, M. E.; Le, G.-W. Millets: nutritional composition, some health benefits and processing – a review. Food Science and Nutrition. Emirate Journal of Food and Agriculture. 2013;25(7):501–508. DOI: 10.9755/ejfa.v25i7.12045

[54] Pack, M.; Hoeler, D.; Lemme, A. Economic assessment of amino acid responses in growing poultry. In: D'Mello, editor. Amino Acids in Animal Nutrition. Wallingford, UK: CAB International; 2003.

[55] Zhang, A.; Liu, X.; Wang, G.; Wang, H.; Liu, J.; Zhao, W.; Zhang, Y. Crude fat content and fatty acid profile and their correlations in foxtail millet. Cereal Chemistry. 2015;92(5):455–459. DOI: 10.1094/CCHEM-12-14-0252-R

[56] Zambiazi, R. C.; Przybylski, R.; Weber Zambiazi, M.;, Barbosa Mendoca, C. Fatty acid composition of vegetable oils and fats. B. CEPPA, Curitiba. 2007;25(1):111–120.

[57] Nakayama, H.; Afzal, M.; Okuno, K. Intraspecific differentiation and geographical distribution of Wx alleles for low amylose content in endosperm of foxtail millet (*Setaria italica* L.) Beauv. Euphytica. 1998;102(3):289–293. DOI: 10.1023/A:1018344819531

[58] Zhu, F. Review. Structure, physicochemical properties, and uses of millet starch. Food Research International. 2014;64:200–211. DOI: 10.1016/j.foodres.2014.06.026

[59] Saleh, A. S. M.; Zhankg, Q.; Chen, J.; Shen, Q. Millet grains: nutritional quality, processing, and potential health benefits. Comprehensive Reviews in Food Science and Food Safety. 2013;12:281–295.

[60] Zhang, L. Z.; Liu, R. H. Phenolic and carotenoid profiles and antiproliferative activity of foxtail millet. Food Chemistry. 2015;174:495–501. DOI: 10.1016/j.foodchem.2014.09.089

[61] AU: Please provide English translation of text instead of other language in Ref. [61].Hermuth, J. Čirok znovu vzkříšená plodina v ČR. Agromanuál. 2010;5:62–65 (in Czech).

[62] AU: Please provide volume number for Ref. [62].Martin, J. H.; MacMasters, M. M. Industrial uses for grain sorghum. USDA Yearbook 1950–51. 1952:349–352.

[63] Martin, J. H.; Waldren, R. P.; Stamp, D. L. Principles of Field Crop Production. Upper Saddle River, NJ: Pearson/Prentice Hall; 2006. p. 954.

[64] Jambunathan, R.; Subramainian, V. Grain quality and utilisation of sorghum and pearl millet. In: Biotechnology Workshop; 12–15 January 1988; Pantacheru, India: ICRISAT; 1988. p. 133–139.

[65] AU: Please provide English translation of text instead of other language in Ref. [65]. Also provide volume number for the same.Zeman, L. Katalog krmiv. Brno. 1991:191 (in Czech).

[66] Mosse, J.; Huet, J.-C.; Baudet, J. The amino acid composition of whole sorghum grain in relation to its nitrogen content. Cereal Chemistry. 1988;65(4):271–277.

[67] Matz, S. A. Other cereal grains. In: Matz, S. A., editors. The Chemistry and Technology of Cereals as Food and Feed. 2nd ed. Westport: The AVI Publishing Company; 1991. p. 259–284.

[68] Serna-Saldiva, R. S.; Rooney, L. W. Structure and chemistry of sorghum and millets. In: Dendy, D. A. V., editor. Sorghum and Millets. Chemistry and Technology. St. Paul, Minnesota: Am. Assoc. of Cereal Chemists; 1995. p. 69–124.

[69] AU: Please provide English translation of text instead of other language in Ref. [69].Ivanišová, E. Biologicky cenné zložky obilnín a pseudoobilnín. Agromagazín. 2009;10:18–22 (in Slovak).

[70] AU: Please provide English translation of text instead of other language in Ref. [70].Podrábský, M. Nový hybrid čiroku se súdánskou trávou. Agromanuál. 2008;3:36–37 (in Czech).

[71] AU: Please provide publisher location for Ref. [71].Bolsen, K. K.; Moore, K. J.; Coblentz, W. K.; Siefers, M. K.; White J. S. Sorghum silage. In: Silage Science and Technology. American Society of Agronomy Inc., Crop Science Society of America Inc, Soil Science Society of America Inc.; 2003. p. 609–632.

[72] Habyarimana, E.; Laureti, D.; De Ninno, M. C.; Lorenzoni, C. Performances of biomass sorghum [Sorghum bicolor (L.) Moench] under different water regimes in Mediterranean region. Industrial Crops and Products. 2004;20:23–28. DOI: doi:10.1016/j.indcrop.2003.12.019

[73] Windpassingera, S.; Friedta, W.; Frauenb, M.; Snowdona, R.; Wittkopa, B. Designing adapted sorghum silage types with an enhanced energy density for biogas generation in temperate Europe. Biomass and Bioenergy. 2015;81:496–504. DOI: 10.1016/j.biombioe.2015.08.005

[74] Chynoweth, D. P.; Turick, C. E.; Owens, J. M.; Jerger, D. E.; Peck, M. W. Biochemical methane potential of biomass and waste feedstocks. Biomass and Bioenergy. 1993;5(1): 95–111.

[75] Amon, T.; Amon, B.; Kryvoruchko, V.; Zollitsch, W.; Mayer, K.; Gruber, L. Biogas production from maize and dairy cattle manure-influence of biomass composition on the methane yield. Agriculture, Ecosystems and Environment. 2007;118(1–4):173–182. DOI: 10.1016/j.agee.2006.05.007

[76] Mahmood, A.; Honermeier, B. Chemical composition and methane yield of sorghum cultivars with contrasting row spacing. Field Crops Research. 2012;128:27–33. DOI: 10.1016/j.fcr.2011.12.010

Chapter 2

Ulva Genus as Alternative Crop: Nutritional and Functional Properties

Jesús Alberto Vázquez-Rodríguez and
Carlos Abel Amaya-Guerra

Additional information is available at the end of the chapter

http://dx.doi.org/10.5772/62787

Abstract

Use of seaweed by humans is an ancient practice. In Asian countries, the use of them in human and animal feed, traditional medicine, and compost in agriculture is well documented. Since the twenty-first century begins, the scientific interest for seaweed had increased in Occidental countries. *Ulva* or *Enteromorpha* is a green macroalgae genus that raises and cultivates around the world. It has salinity tolerance and growth with diverse nitrogen ratios, be able to farm them in aquaculture systems. Scientific studies seen in this genus an interesting profile of chemical compounds: The protein is similar in quantity and quality to soy or some animal products; dietetic fiber percentage is elevated (>40%), being around 40% soluble fiber of them. In addition, fiber fraction presents Ulvan, a complex sulfated polysaccharide that presents antiviral, antihyperlipidemic, and antidiabetic effect in animal assays. Moreover, antioxidant and phytochemical profile has not being totally elucidated, giving important opportunities to scientific community for explode consciously this biological resource.

Keywords: *Ulva* , *Enteromorpha* , algae, Ulvan, functional food

1. Introduction

For centuries, food has been used to promote health, but the knowledge of the relationship between food components and health is now being understanding, helping to improve food quality or discover new nutrient sources. Use of seaweed in human and animal feed, as natural medicine, is a practice that goes back many eras, mainly in Asian countries. In Occident, mostly they had been confined as raw material for obtaining phycocolloids. Since the twenty-first century initiates, the innovation of algae as a crop, predominantly *Ulva* species had made an increase in the possible uses in food and health industry. The evidence had showed *Ulva* species present agronomical and nutritional facts scientifically interesting. The *Ulva* genus is tolerant to environmental challenges, and the biomass increases in fast way. Nutritionally, the protein ratio is similar to some legumes and some varieties shown high digestibility (>90%). The lipid fraction contains polyunsaturated fatty acids (PUFA) and another fatty compounds of interest, as alpha linoleic acid (ALA). However, fiber fraction and antioxidant compounds would be the most interesting elements; which present antioxidant activity, support to decrease glucose, cholesterol, and triglycerides levels in blood, among other benefic health effects. The aim of this chapter is to review about *Ulva* as an alternative crop and its role as functional food and nutraceutical compounds source.

2. Biological characteristics of *Ulva*

The employment of seaweeds in human and animal nutrition had been practiced for centuries, principally in Oriental countries, mainly in China, Japan, and South Asia area. In the last decades, European and American countries as France, Scotland, Peru, and Chile had been added this crop as ingredient in traditional food [1]. However, the most part of the seaweed species founded in littoral areas around the world is used as a basis in phycocolloides extraction, utilized in textile, chemistry, and food industry; or as agronomic basis for fertilizes [2].

One cosmopolite green seaweed group is Ulvaceae family. The genus *Ulva* (subsequently denominated *Ulva* in text) has specific biological and physiological characteristics. *Ulva* frequently is distributed marine environment with its few freshwater representatives, with variation of salinity, temperature, water quality, and grow successfully in nutrient-rich habitats [3, 4]. Macroscopically shape is filament-like and membranous (leaf-like), growing in form of typical vividly green tube- or leaf-shaped thalli, o en also with various types of branches, attached to the substrate by rhizoids, or later as free-floating intestinoid clusters [5]. *Ulva* forms morphologically similar haploid and diploid thalli, both of which produce asexual zoospores by mitotic division of vegetative cells [6], showing biflagellate or quadriflagellate gametes or zoospores. In addition, the cell has complex and thick cell wall made of microfibrils with irregular settled; containing one parietal and cup-shaped chloroplast with one or numerous pyrenoids [6, 7]. For these reasons, taxonomically *Ulva* is complicated macroalgal group and usually confused with *Enteromorpha* genus; they are used as synonyms. If the differentiation of both genus is required, it would be necessary genetic and/or ultrastructure studies [8].

2.1. *Ulva* as a crop: agronomical uses and advantages

Ulva is widely distributed around the world and tolerant to some environmental challenges, enabling the amount of biomass generated being in order of tons. Around 16 million tons of seaweeds (fresh weight basis) and other marine plants are annually produced or collected with an estimated value of 5575 million Euros worldwide [9]; at the same time, seaweeds are currently considered as an underexploited or barely not exploited natural resource [10–12]. In a Mexican report, the biomass generated by *Ulva* in Golfo de México littoral had been quantified, showing around 360–426 ton weight dry basis, mostly of them, being wasted or eliminated [13], due the deoxygenation of water and fish deaths, besides the unsightly and undesirable odor when in decomposition [14].

Most of the metric tons of seaweed are used as nutrient supplement or biostimulant/biofertilizer to increase plant growth and yield. Studies have revealed a wide range of beneficial effects of seaweed extract applications on agronomic plantation; helping to improve agriculture practices as seed germination, performance yield and decrease stress, and upgrade postharvest shelf-life of unpreserved products [11]. Seaweed components such as macroelement and microelement nutrients, amino acids, vitamins, cytokinins, auxins, and abscisic acid (ABA)—such as growth substances affect cellular metabolism in treated plants leading to enhanced growth and crop yield [15–17], but many of the action modes or biochemical pathways activated are unknown or barely elucidated [11].

Literature mentioned that *Ulva* contains some metabolites and polysaccharides would act as effective elicitors of plant defense against plant diseases. A study using extracts of *Ulva* spp. against *Colletotrichum trifolii* in *Medicago truncatula* showed disease resistance without the elicitation of necrotic lesions [18]. *Ulva* extract elicited the expression of the PR-10 gene. The PR-10 gene belongs to the group of pathogenesis-related genes (PR) important for active defense against diseases following pathogen attack [19], be able to up regulate until 152 genes related to plant defense [18].

As its know, the different algae species present alginates and another complex polysaccharides which retain water and minerals, helping to moisture and growing of plants. A mix of salts of alginic acid and metallic ions in the soil helps to absorb moisture and make and swelling effect, intensification mud structure, making a healthier soil for plant root system [20].

In other hand, cultivate seaweed, as *Ulva* could be a form to reduce aquaculture pollution, generating biomass utilizable for another industries. The aquaculture industry, predominantly land-based aquaculture, generates more than 65 million tons of organisms cultivated annually [9]. The intensive aquaculture production is reliant on high-protein feed to facilitate the rapid growth of animals. Nevertheless, the protein conversion ratio of aquatic organisms is relatively ineffective, resulting in nutrient-rich remaining [21]. If released directly into the environment, these waste nutrients can cause significant environmental degradation through nitrogen enrichment and lead to the proliferation of algal growth [22], producing an unbalance in oxygenation of water.

Seaweeds as *Ulva* can be cultivated in aquaculture wastewater to recover a high proportion of these waste nutrients, while simultaneously creating a biomass resource [23]. The integration of seaweed cultivation with land-based aquaculture for nutrient remediation has been successfully demonstrated at a research level numerous times [23–25], although rarely implemented commercially [26]. One of the major reasons for this is that the seaweed biomass produced requires a market, or on-site use; otherwise, the seaweed biomass itself can become a waste product and liability [27].

One of the lowest cost approaches to explode this biomass is composting, which is the aerobic decomposition of organic material by successive microbial communities. To successfully compost any organic waste, the carbon-to-nitrogen ratio of the material needs to be balanced. As seaweed is a relatively novel feedstock for composting, it is unknown as to how the initial C:N ratio of seaweed-based composts will influence the composting process and the quality of the mature compost, but studies had demonstrated that it is feasible, making a high-quality compost, with C:N ratio for seaweed-based composts to be 22:1, which corresponds to seaweed accounting for 82% of the compost on a fresh weight basis [27]. Another way of decrease nutrient waste in aquaculture by *Ulva* culture is through fluid systems, making possible remove total N in water, increasing optical transmittance of light [28]. Additionally, *Ulva* methanolic extract presents antialgal activity against red tide microalgae [29], which could act as biological contaminant in aquaculture.

2.2. Nutritional evidences of *Ulva* algae

At the same time, as food has long been used to improve health, our knowledge of the relationship between food components and health is now being used to improve food [30]. The foods that provide nutrients and additionally promote health had been denominated "functional food". Functional foods can provide health benefits by reducing the risk of chronic diseases and enhancing the ability to manage chronic diseases, thus improving the quality of life. Functional foods also can promote growth and development and enhance performance [30].

Seaweeds have become a valuable vegetable, fresh or dried, and an important food ingredient in the human diet [31], mainly in Oriental countries and lately in European and Latin American countries. They are identifiable by present protein, polysaccharides, mineral, and some vitamins in important percentages.

Interest in *Ulva* as a "newness food" is expanding in Western countries. The nutritional information about *Ulva* has been focused in: *Ulva lactuca, Ulva pertusa, Ulva fasciata, Ulva rigida, Enteromorpha* sp., *Enteromorpha flexuosa, Enteromorpha intestinalis,* and *Enteromorpha compressa* [32].

Normally, the chemical composition of *Ulva* has 9–14% protein; 2–3.6% ether extract (n-3 and n-6 fatty acids 10.4 and 10.9 g/100 g of total fatty acid); 32–36% ash. Alkaloids, cyanogenic

Ulva species	Protein (%)	Lipid (%)	Ash (%)	Total dietetic fiber (%)	Insoluble fiber (%)	Soluble fiber (%)
Ulva spp. (as *Enteromorpha* spp.) [33]	9.45–14.10	2.20–3.60	32.64–36.38	–	–	–
Ulva clathrata [34]	13.13	2.92	18.36	44.44	–	–
Ulva clathrata [32]	21.9–26.9	2.5–3.5	44.8–49.6	24.8–26.3	8.7–10.7	15.6–16.6
Ulva lactuca [35]	8.46	7.87	19.59	54.90	34.27	20.53
Ulva spp. [30]	7–44	0.3–1.6	11–55	38	17	21
Ulva lactuca [36]	7.06	1.64	21.3	55.4	–	–

Table 1. Chemical composition of *Ulva* species

glucids, saponins, and tannic acid are near to null [33]. In **Table 1**, some *Ulva* species are titled by nutritional characteristics.

2.3. Protein of Ulvales: amino acidic profile and bioactive peptides

The protein ratio of Ulvales would oscillate by different factors, as the species is cultivated or marine source, changes in seasonal periods [31], principally. Generally, the highest protein value has been found during the period of winter–early spring and the lowest during summer–early autumn [37].

Diverse researchers had found interesting information about the *Ulva* protein, presenting an amino acidic profile comparable to soy or another legumes, peptides with bioactivity against inflammation processes, antivirals, among others. *Ulva* founded in Mexican littorals was analyzed, and the results for amino acids content shown 9 of the 10 considered essential for humans are present in protein of *Ulva* spp., a higher quantity than in an equivalent weight of soy [33]. The concentration of isoleucine, leucine, lysine, and threonine is higher to the FAO-OMS pattern [38]. Protein digestibility by enzymatic assay was 98% compared to the reference casein pattern. Anti-nutritional factors (tannins, alkaloids, cyanogenic glucids, and saponin) that could affect digestibility were scarce to none [33].

In Hong Kong and Tunisia areas had been reported similar results about amino acids for *Ulva*. The essential amino acid score analysis of *U. lactuca* shown seaweed samples contained all the essential amino acids (in different proportions, excluding tryptophan), which accounted for 42.1 ± 48.4% of the total amino acid content, being Leucine was limiting amino acid but to be able to contribute adequate levels of total EAA [35, 36]. *Ulva armoricana* contains high levels of the amino acid proline (approximately 5–11%) of total amino acids, while *U. pertusa* is reported to have an arginine content of 15% [39, 40].

For these reasons, *Ulva* protein had been used by the fortification in some reports. The results for bread shown that an *Ulva* and *Cladophora* spp. mixture increases the protein percentage with minimal variations in sensory and technological properties [14]. In case of maize tortilla, the protein percentage was significantly increased but in chemical compute, the *Ulva* protein was not complementary to maize protein. The rheological and sensorial properties in maize tortilla were slightly modified [34]. In addition, the free amino acid fraction of seaweed is mainly composed of alanine, arginine, aspartic, and glutamic acid; given the characteristic taste of "sea product" [34, 41] (**Table 2**).

A myriad of positive health beneficial properties is associated with bioactive peptides including antihypertensive, anti-diabetic, anti-obesity, immune-modulatory, relaxing, and satiety-inducing effects [42]. Bioactive peptides used as functional food ingredients do not accumulate in body tissue, and there are only a few reports regarding negative side effects when bioactive peptides are used for preventative healthcare purposes. In the case of *Ulva* genus had been isolated a mitogenic hexapeptide, SECMA 1. This peptide was shown to be involved in the modulation of cell proliferation-associated molecules, proteoglycans and glycosaminoglycans in human foreskin fibroblasts [43].

Amino acid	*Ulva* spp. flour
Taurine	0.09
Hydroxiproline	0.34
Aspartic acid	1.70
Threonine	0.71
Serine	0.69
Glutamic acid	1.73
Proline	0.50
Lantionine	0.02
Glycine	0.85
Alanine	1.28
Cysteine	0.30
Valine	0.80
Methionine	0.26
Isoleucine	0.48
Leucine	0.75
Tyrosine	0.31
Phenylalanine	0.64
Hydroxilysine	0.18
Ornithine	0.12
Lysine	0.48
Hystidine	0.12
Arginine	0.68
Tryptophan	0.10
Total	13.13
Protein crude (N × 6.25) grams	14.99

*Grams per 100 g sample. Extracted with the permission from Vázquez Rodríguez et al [34].

Table 2. Amino acids profile of *Ulva* spp.

In addition, *Ulva* presents bioactive lectins. These proteins interact with specific glycan structures, making glycoconjugates. The protein–carbohydrate interaction is responsible for participation in numerous biological and immunological processes [44]. Furthermore, lectin has been found to increase the agglutination of blood cells (erythrocytes) and is also useful in the detection of disease-related alterations of glycan synthesis, including infectious agents such as viruses, bacteria, fungi, and parasites [10, 45, 46]. Other bioactive properties exhibited by marine algal lectins include antibiotic, mitogenic, cytotoxic, anti-nociceptive, anti-inflammatory, anti-adhesion, and anti-HIV activities [45, 47, 48].

2.4. Dietary fiber in *Ulva*: Ulvan as bioactive polymer

Dietetic fiber is a complex mixture of polysaccharides no digestible. Structurally, polysaccharides are polymers of simple sugars (monosaccharides) linked together by glycosidic bonds, and this characteristic gives them numerous commercial applications in products such as stabilizers, thickeners, emulsifiers, and generally, food industry. The total polysaccharide concentrations in the seaweed species of interest range from 4 to 76% of dry weight; in *Ulva* species, the concentration would be until 65% of dry weight [9].

In algae, the cell wall polysaccharides mainly consist of cellulose and hemicelluloses, neutral polysaccharides, and are thought to physically support the thallus in water. The cellulose and hemicellulose content of *Ulva* species is around 9% both. Lignin is characteristic of *Ulva* sp., with concentrations of 3% dry weight [49]. As storage polysaccharides, green algae contain sulfuric acid polysaccharides, sulfated galactans, and xylans [30].

The seaweed dietary fibers contain some valuable nutrients and substances, and there has been a deal of interest in seaweed meal, functional foods, and nutraceuticals for human consumption by the presence of complex polysaccharides; shown antitumor and antiherpetitic bioactivity; they are potent as an anticoagulant and decrease low-density lipid (LDL)-cholesterols in rats (hypercholesterolemia); they prevent obesity, large intestine cancer, and diabetes; and they have antiviral activities [46, 50–54]. Moreover, glucose availability and absorption are delayed in the proximal small intestine after the addition of soluble fibers, thus reducing postprandial glucose levels [55]. Water-insoluble polysaccharides are mainly associated with a decrease in digestive tract transit time [41].

In the green algae, most work has focused on storage polysaccharides. In *Ulva* genus, these are known as Ulvan. Ulvan and derives display several biological activities of potential interest for therapeutic, nutraceutical, and personal care applications [42]. Ulvans are highly sulfated polysaccharides (189–8200 kDa [56]) composed by a mix of rhamnose, uronic acid, and xylose as the main monomers. Furthermore, the Ulvans containing a disaccharide, the aldobiuronic acid, [→4)-D-glucuronic acid-(1→4)-L-rhamnose3-sulphate-(1→], and iduronic acid. As dietary fiber, Ulvans contain a water-soluble fraction and insoluble material, similar to cellulose.

The mechanism of gel formation of Ulvan is exceptional between polysaccharide hydrogels and phycocolloids. The Ulvan rheology is compared with Arabic gum but presents another characteristics not fully understood due to its physicochemical interactions are very complex. Ulvans have thermoreversible behavior without thermal hysteresis, and its gelling properties are affected by boric acid, divalent cations as Ca^{+} and pH. These properties perhaps of interest for chelating application [30, 56], among others.

These properties make to Ulvans highly water absorbent and under some conditions, biodegradable hydrocolloid; making desirable for some industries. Relationally to food industry, Ulvans can constitute an effective and low-cost alternative to meat-derived products because their rheological and gelling properties make them suitable substitutes for gelatin and related compounds [57].

Medical and pharmacologically, Ulvans and their oligosaccharides present anticoagulant, antioxidant, antiviral, anticancer, and immunomodulation activities [12]. They were able to modify the adhesion and proliferation of normal and tumoral human colonic cells as well as the expression of transforming growth factors and surface glycosyl markers related to cellular differentiation [58]. Ulvan is rich in iduronic acid. Iduronic acid is used in the synthesis of heparin fragment analogues with anti-thrombotic activities [56]. Oligosaccharides from *Ulva* could be used as reference compounds for analyzing biologically active domains of glycosaminoglycan-like heparin [59]. Ulvans possess immune-modulatory activities that may be of potential application in stimulating the immune response or controlling immune cell activity to mitigate associated negative effects, such as inflammation. It had been proved that low-Mw sulfated Ulvans from *U. lactuca* and their desulfated derivatives have anticancer activities because they can inhibit Caco-2 cell proliferation and/or differentiation in cell culture tests [60]. In reports had evaluated the effects of a water-soluble acidic polysaccharide from *U. rigida* on the activities of RAW264.7 murine macrophages. However, these effects considerably decreased after desulfation of the polysaccharides, which suggests that the sulfate group is essential for the stimulatory capacity of these molecules [61].

Furthermore, Ulvans present antiviral effects. Some research indicates that almost all Ulvan fractions from *E. compressa* shown potent anti-HSV-1 activity as well as low cytotoxicity to host cells [62]. Extracts from *U. lactuca* can inhibit Japanese encephalitis virus (JEV) infection in Vero cells because the SP can block JEV adsorption and thus hinder the entry of JEV into the cells [63].

Much of the characteristics mentioned before are due to antioxidant activity present in Ulvans. Ulvans have emerged as prospective candidates for effective, nontoxic substances [64, 65] with potent antioxidant activity [66, 67] because they generally act as free-radical inhibitors or scavengers and, therefore, primary antioxidants. These effects include superoxide radical scavenging, hydroxyl radical scavenging, DPPH (1,1-diphenyl-2-picrylhydrazyl) radical scavenging, total antioxidant capacity, power reducing ability, and ferrous chelating ability. However, in terms of antioxidant potential, some crude Ulvans show effects no greater than those from red or brown algae (carrageenan and fucoidan) [68]. Even that the enzymatic or chemical digestion of Ulvans is adept; obtaining in some cases, fractions with anti-hyperlipidemic effects [69] and a significantly effect of sulfated degree in antioxidant and quelant effect [70]. Ulvans from *U. pertusa* also show antihyperlipidemic activity, affecting total cholesterol and LDL-cholesterol in blood serum [71]. The causal mechanisms of this bioactivity are unclear, but bile acid sequestration is hypothesized [69]. Additionally, the particular chemical structure of Ulvan make complicated fermentation process by colonic bacterial [72].

The commercial limitation of Ulvan and dietetic fiber of *Ulva* is based in its diverse and complex structure [73, 74], making difficult the standardization of properties [52, 62, 68, 75–77]; and the fiber fraction, mainly the insoluble fraction, quelate lead and another heavy metals, highly toxic to human or another animals, due to its extraction and use should be managed with quality control measures [35].

2.5. *Ulva* as a source of phytochemicals: bioactivity and nutraceutical function

Many studies already demonstrated the promising properties of macroalgae extracts, as health promoters. Anticoagulant, anti-proliferative, antiviral, antimicrobial, among others bioactivities are some of his characteristics. Notwithstanding macroalgae are known to contain numerous phytochemicals such as terpenes, phenolics, sterols, vitamins, principally. Their detailed chemical characterization and the identification of bioactive action are still largely unexplored in many species [78].

For example, the lipoid fraction of *Ulva* is slightly minor than protein or fiber fractions, but the fatty acid compounds presents in their make it relevant. Some researchers had found in *U. lactuca* numerous fatty acids (saturated and unsaturated) and relative compounds as diacids, long-chain aliphatic alcohols, sterols, monoglycerides, diterpenes, and tocopheroles; all valuable lipophilic components with well-established nutritional and health benefits [78].

Ethanolic extract of *U. rigida* (4.31 ± 0.74 μmol gallic acid g-1) presented anti-hyperglycemic, anti-oxidative, and genotoxic/antigenotoxic capacity *in vivo* in diabetic mellitus-induced rats. The possible mechanisms by which *U. rigida* exerts its antihyperglycemic action in diabetic rats may be due to the regeneration of b-cells in the islets of pancreas and/or potentiating the insulin release [79]. *U. rigida* presents a vast quantity of antioxidant as chlorophyll a, b, carotenoids, vitamins A, C, and E, phenolic content, among others; all them with important bioactivity [42, 69, 79–82].

Also, *Ulva clathrata* shows an important antioxidant potential in comparison with other species. This detail could be explained by a high phenolic and flavonoid quantities [83]. The results suggest that these edible green seaweeds possess antioxidant potential which could be considered for future applications in medicine, dietary supplements, cosmetics, or food industries.

3. Conclusions

Ulva genus shows an interesting profile as an alternative crop. Filamentous species of the genus *Ulva* have desirable characteristics for year-round large-scale cultivation, including a broad tolerance of salinity and temperature with high growth rates, enabling production in enclosed and open waters. Relatedly to human and/or animal nutrition, *Ulva* presents a balance of nutrients, as protein with amino score similar to legume or animal protein, an important PUFA fraction, dietetic fiber with functional activity (technological and nutritionally); furthermore of an important presence of various antioxidants as polyphenols, flavonoids, and sulfated compounds, among others, which activate different biochemical pathways, shown beneficial effects to health. In summary, *Ulva* exhibits an interesting agronomic profile and beneficial biological effects, which promotes this alga as an alternative functional crop. Despite the demonstrated properties, the presence of heavy metals should be evaluated, especially lead, for not limiting its use as food or raw material in diverse industries.

Author details

Jesús Alberto Vázquez-Rodríguez[1*] and Carlos Abel Amaya-Guerra[2]

*Address all correspondence to: jesus.vazquezr@uanl.mx

1 Faculty of Public Health and Nutrition, Autonomous University of Nuevo León, Monterrey, México

2 Faculty of Biological Sciences, Autonomous University of Nuevo León, Monterrey, México

References

[1] Zemke-White WL, Ohno M. World seaweed utilisation: An end-of-century summary. J Appl Phycol. 1999;11(4):369–76.

[2] Aguila-Ramírez RN, CJ Hernández-Guerrero, AM Ramírez-Ornelas, A Marín-Álvarez, M Beltrán-López, M Casas-Valdez. Empleo de las algas marinas *Ulva* spp. y *Enteromorpha* spp. en la elaboración de pan. Boletín CICIMAR-IPN. 2002;90:1.

[3] Fletcher RL. The Occurrence of "Green Tides"—A Review. In: Schramm DW, Nienhuis PDPH, editors. Marine Benthic Vegetation [Internet]. Springer: Berlin, Heidelberg; 1996 [cited January 10, 2016]. pp. 7–43. Available from: http://link.springer.com/chapter/10.1007/978-3-642-61398-2_2

[4] Brook AJ, Whitton BA. The Freshwater Algal Flora of the British Isles: An Identification Guide to Freshwater and Terrestrial Algae. In: John DM, editor. Cambridge; New York: Cambridge University Press; 2002. 714 p.

[5] Mareš J. Combined morphological and molecular approach to the assessment of \kur{Ulva} (Chlorophyta, Ulvophyceae) in the Czech Republic [Internet] [Diplomová práce]. University of South Bohemia in České Budějovice, Faculty of Science; 2009 [cited January 10, 2016]. Available from: http://theses.cz/id/v4klp8/?furl=%2Fid%2Fv4klp8%2F;lang=en

[6] Hoek C, Mann D, Jahns HM. Algae: An Introduction to Phycology. Cambridge University Press; 1995. 644 p.

[7] Wehr JD. Freshwater Algae of North America: Ecology and Classification. Academic Press; 2002. 935 p.

[8] Messyasz B, Czerwik-Marcinkowska J, Massalski A, Uher B, Rybak A, Szendzina L, et al. Morphological and ultrastructural studies on *Ulva flexuosa* subsp. pilifera (Chlorophyta) from Poland. Acta Soc Bot Pol. 2013;82(2):157–63.

[9] FAO. FAO Yearbook. Fishery and Aquaculture Statistics. 2012 [Internet]. 2012 [cited January 6, 2016]. Available from: http://www.fao.org/3/a-i3740t/index.html

[10] Cardozo KHM, Guaratini T, Barros MP, Falcão VR, Tonon AP, Lopes NP, et al. Metabolites from algae with economical impact. Comp Biochem Physiol Part C Toxicol Pharmacol. 2007;146(1–2):60–78.

[11] Khan W, Rayirath UP, Subramanian S, Jithesh MN, Rayorath P, Hodges DM, et al. Seaweed extracts as biostimulants of plant growth and development. J Plant Growth Regul. 2009;28(4):386–99.

[12] Jiménez-Escrig A, Gómez-Ordóñez E, Rupérez P. Chapter 26—Seaweed as a Source of Novel Nutraceuticals: Sulfated Polysaccharides and Peptides. In: Se-Kwon Kim, editor. Advances in Food and Nutrition Research [Internet]. Academic Press; 2011 [cited January 8, 2013]. pp. 325–37. Available from: http://www.sciencedirect.com/science/article/pii/B9780123876690000260

[13] Pacheco-Ruíz I, Zertuche-González JA, Chee-Barragán A, Arroyo-Ortega E. Biomass and potential commercial utilization of *Ulva lactuca* (Chlorophyta, Ulvaceae) beds along the north-west coast of the Gulf of California. Phycologia. 2002;41(2):199–201.

[14] Menezes BS, Coelho MS, Meza SLR, Salas-Mellado M, Souza MRAZ. Macroalgal biomass as an additional ingredient of bread. Int Food Res J. 2015;22(2):812–7.

[15] Durand N, Briand X, Meyer C. The effect of marine bioactive substances (N PRO) and exogenous cytokinins on nitrate reductase activity in *Arabidopsis thaliana*. Physiol Plant. 2003;119(4):489–93.

[16] Stirk WA, Novák O, Strnad M, Staden J van. Cytokinins in macroalgae. Plant Growth Regul. 2003;41(1):13–24.

[17] Ördög V, Stirk WA, Van Staden J, Novák O, Strnad M. Endogenous cytokinins in three genera of microalgae from the chlorophyta1. J Phycol. 2004;40(1):88–95.

[18] Cluzet S, Torregrosa C, Jacquet C, Lafitte C, Fournier J, Mercier L, et al. Gene expression profiling and protection of *Medicago truncatula* against a fungal infection in response to an elicitor from green algae *Ulva* spp. Plant Cell Environ. 2004;27(7):917–28.

[19] Loon LC van, Rep M, Pieterse CMJ. Significance of inducible defense-related proteins in infected plants. Annu Rev Phytopathol. 2006;44(1):135–62.

[20] Gandhiyappan K, Perumal P. Growth promoting effect of seaweed liquid fertilizer (*Enteromorpha intestinalis*) on the sesame crop plant. Seaweed Resour Util. 2001;23:23–5.

[21] Crab R, Avnimelech Y, Defoirdt T, Bossier P, Verstraete W. Nitrogen removal techniques in aquaculture for a sustainable production. Aquaculture. 2007;270(1–4):1–14.

[22] Anderson DM, Cembella AD, Hallegraeff GM. Progress in understanding harmful algal blooms: Paradigm shifts and new technologies for research, monitoring, and management. Annu Rev Mar Sci. 2012;4(1):143–76.

[23] Mata L, Schuenhoff A, Santos R. A direct comparison of the performance of the seaweed biofilters, *Asparagopsis armata* and *Ulva rigida*. J Appl Phycol. 2010;22(5):639–44.

[24] Neori A, Msuya FE, Shauli L, Schuenhoff A, Kopel F, Shpigel M. A novel three-stage seaweed (*Ulva lactuca*) biofilter design for integrated mariculture. J Appl Phycol. 2003;15(6):543–53.

[25] Msuya FE, Neori A. Effect of water aeration and nutrient load level on biomass yield, N uptake and protein content of the seaweed *Ulva lactuca* cultured in seawater tanks. J Appl Phycol. 2008;20(6):1021–31.

[26] Bolton JJ, Robertson-Andersson DV, Shuuluka D, Kandjengo L. Growing *Ulva* (Chlorophyta) in integrated systems as a commercial crop for abalone feed in South Africa: A SWOT analysis. J Appl Phycol. 2008;21(5):575–83.

[27] Cole AJ, Roberts DA, Garside AL, Nys R de, Paul NA. Seaweed compost for agricultural crop production. J Appl Phycol. 2015;1–14.

[28] Hadley S, Wild-Allen K, Johnson C, Macleod C. Modeling macroalgae growth and nutrient dynamics for integrated multi-trophic aquaculture. J Appl Phycol. 2014;27(2): 901–16.

[29] Ying-ying S, Hui W, Gan-lin G, Yin-fang P, Bin-lun Y, Chang-hai W. Green alga *Ulva pertusa*—A new source of bioactive compounds with antialgal activity. Environ Sci Pollut Res. 2015;22(13):10351–9.

[30] Holdt SL, Kraan S. Bioactive compounds in seaweed: Functional food applications and legislation. J Appl Phycol. 2011;23(3):543–97.

[31] Fleurence J. Seaweed proteins: Biochemical, nutritional aspects and potential uses. Trends Food Sci Technol. 1999;10(1):25–8.

[32] Peña-Rodríguez A, Mawhinney TP, Ricque-Marie D, Cruz-Suárez LE. Chemical composition of cultivated seaweed *Ulva clathrata* (Roth) C. Agardh. Food Chem. 2011;129(2):491–8.

[33] Aguilera-Morales M, Casas-Valdez M, Carrillo-Domínguez S, González-Acosta B, Pérez-Gil F. Chemical composition and microbiological assays of marine algae *Enteromorpha* spp. as a potential food source. J Food Compos Anal. 2005;18(1):79–88.

[34] Vázquez Rodríguez JA. Desarrollo de tortillas de maíz fortificadas con fuentes de proteína y fibra y su efecto biológico en un modelo animal [Tesis Doctoral]. [Nuevo León, México]: Universidad Autónoma de Nuevo León; 2013.

[35] Yaich H, Garna H, Besbes S, Paquot M, Blecker C, Attia H. Chemical composition and functional properties of *Ulva lactuca* seaweed collected in Tunisia. Food Chem. 2011;128(4):895–901.

[36] Wong KH, Cheung PCK. Nutritional evaluation of some subtropical red and green seaweeds: Part I—Proximate composition, amino acid profiles and some physico-chemical properties. Food Chem. 2000;71(4):475–82.

[37] Galland-Irmouli AV, Fleurence J, Lamghari R, Luçon M, Rouxel C, Barbaroux O, . Nutritional value of proteins from edible seaweed *Palmaria palmata* (dulse). J Nutr Biochem. 1999;10(6):353–9.

[38] Young VR. Adult Amino Acid Requirements: The case for a major revision in current recommendations. J Nutr. 1994;124(8 Suppl):1517S–23S.

[39] Fujiwara-Arasaki T, Mino N, Kuroda M. The Protein Value in Human Nutrition of Edible Marine Algae in Japan. In: Bird CJ, Ragan MA, editors. Eleventh International Seaweed Symposium [Internet]. Springer: Netherlands; 1984 [cited January 11, 2016]. pp. 513–6. Available from: http://link.springer.com/chapter/10.1007/978-94-009-6560-7_104

[40] Fleurence J, Coeur CL, Mabeau S, Maurice M, Landrein A. Comparison of different extractive procedures for proteins from the edible seaweeds *Ulva rigida* and *Ulva rotundata*. J Appl Phycol. 1995;7(6):577–82.

[41] Mabeau S, Fleurence J. Seaweed in food products: biochemical and nutritional aspects. Trends Food Sci Technol. 1993;4(4):103–7.

[42] Hayes M, Tiwari BK. Bioactive carbohydrates and peptides in foods: An overview of sources, downstream processing steps and associated bioactivities. Int J Mol Sci. 2015;16(9):22485–508.

[43] Ennamany R, Saboureau D, Mekideche N, Creppy EE. SECMA 1, a mitogenic hexapeptide from *Ulva* algeae modulates the production of proteoglycans and glycosaminoglycans in human foreskin fibroblast. Hum Exp Toxicol. 1998;17(1):18–22.

[44] Hori K, Matsubara K, Miyazawa K. Primary structures of two hemagglutinins from the marine red alga, Hypnea japonica1. Biochim Biophys Acta BBA Gen Subj. 2000;1474(2):226–36.

[45] Bird KT, Chiles TC, Longley RE, Kendrick AF, Kinkema MD. Agglutinins from marine macroalgae of the southeastern United States. J Appl Phycol. 1993;5(2):213–8.

[46] Murata M, Nakazoe J. Production and Use of Marine Algae in Japan. JARQ Jpn [Internet]. 2001 [cited January 11, 2016]; Available from: http://agris.fao.org/agris-search/search.do?recordID=JP2002003712

[47] Mori J, Matsunaga T, Takahashi S, Hasegawa C, Saito H. Inhibitory activity on lipid peroxidation of extracts from marine brown alga. Phytother Res. 2003;17(5):549–51.

[48] Smit AJ. Medicinal and pharmaceutical uses of seaweed natural products: A review. J Appl Phycol. 2004;16(4):245–62.

[49] Marinho-Soriano E, Fonseca PC, Carneiro MAA, Moreira WSC. Seasonal variation in the chemical composition of two tropical seaweeds. Bioresour Technol. 2006;97(18):2402–6.

[50] Lee J-B, Hayashi K, Hashimoto M, Nakano T, Hayashi T. Novel antiviral fucoidan from sporophyll of *Undaria pinnatifida* (Mekabu). Chem Pharm Bull (Tokyo). 2004;52(9): 1091–4.

[51] Amano H, Kakinuma M, Coury DA, Ohno H, Hara T. Effect of a seaweed mixture on serum lipid level and platelet aggregation in rats. Fish Sci. 2005;71(5):1160–6.

[52] Athukorala Y, Lee K-W, Kim S-K, Jeon Y-J. Anticoagulant activity of marine green and brown algae collected from Jeju Island in Korea. Bioresour Technol. 2007;98(9):1711–6.

[53] Ghosh T, Chattopadhyay K, Marschall M, Karmakar P, Mandal P, Ray B. Focus on antivirally active sulfated polysaccharides: From structure–activity analysis to clinical evaluation. Glycobiology. 2009;19(1):2–15.

[54] Ye H, Wang K, Zhou C, Liu J, Zeng X. Purification, antitumor and antioxidant activities in vitro of polysaccharides from the brown seaweed *Sargassum pallidum*. Food Chem. 2008;111(2):428–32.

[55] Jenkins DJ, Wolever TM, Leeds AR, Gassull MA, Haisman P, Dilawari J, . Dietary fibres, fibre analogues, and glucose tolerance: Importance of viscosity. Br Med J. 1978;1(6124): 1392–4.

[56] Lahaye M, Inizan F, Vigoureux J. NMR analysis of the chemical structure of Ulvan and of Ulvan-boron complex formation. Carbohydr Polym. 1998;36(2–3):239–49.

[57] Choi YS, Hong SR, Lee YM, Song KW, Park MH, Nam YS. Study on gelatin-containing artificial skin: I. Preparation and characteristics of novel gelatin-alginate sponge. Biomaterials. 1999;20(5):409–17.

[58] Lahaye M, Robic A. Structure and functional properties of Ulvan, a polysaccharide from green seaweeds. Biomacromolecules. 2007;8(6):1765–74.

[59] Paradossi G, Cavalieri F, Chiessi E. A conformational study on the algal polysaccharide Ulvan†. Macromolecules. 2002;35(16):6404–11.

[60] Kaeffer B, Bénard C, Lahaye M, Blottière HM, Cherbut C. Biological properties of Ulvan, a new source of green seaweed sulfated polysaccharides, on cultured normal and cancerous colonic epithelial cells. Planta Med. 1999;65(6):527–31.

[61] Leiro JM, Castro R, Arranz JA, Lamas J. Immunomodulating activities of acidic sulphated polysaccharides obtained from the seaweed *Ulva rigida* C. Agardh. Int Immunopharmacol. 2007;7(7):879–88.

[62] Wang L, Wang X, Wu H, Liu R. Overview on biological activities and molecular characteristics of sulfated polysaccharides from marine green algae in recent years. Mar Drugs. 2014;12(9):4984–5020.

[63] Chiu Y-H, Chan Y-L, Li T-L, Wu C-J. Inhibition of Japanese encephalitis virus infection by the sulfated polysaccharide extracts from *Ulva lactuca*. Mar Biotechnol. 2011;14(4): 468–78.

[64] Alves A, Sousa RA, Reis RL. In vitro cytotoxicity assessment of Ulvan, a polysaccharide extracted from green algae. Phytother Res. 2013;27(8):1143–8.

[65] Rodrigues JAG, Vanderlei E de SO, Araújo IWF de, Quinderé ALG, Coura CO, Benevides NMB. In vivo toxicological evaluation of crude sulfated polysaccharide from the green seaweed *Caulerpa cupressoides* var. lycopodium in Swiss mice. Acta Sci Technol. 2013;35(4):603–10. doi: 10.4025/actascitechnol.v35i4.15699

[66] Batista-Gonzalez AE, Silva AMDOE, Vidal-Novoa A, Pinto JR, Mancini DAP, Mancini-Filho J. Analysis of in vitro and in vivo antioxidant properties of hydrophilic fractions from the seaweed *Halimeda monile* L. J Food Biochem. 2012;36(2):189–97.

[67] Hassan S, El-Twab SA, Hetta M, Mahmoud B. Improvement of lipid profile and antioxidant of hypercholesterolemic albino rats by polysaccharides extracted from the green alga *Ulva lactuca* Linnaeus. Saudi J Biol Sci. 2011;18(4):333–40.

[68] Costa LS, Fidelis GP, Cordeiro SL, Oliveira RM, Sabry DA, Câmara RBG, . Biological activities of sulfated polysaccharides from tropical seaweeds. Biomed Pharmacother. 2010;64(1):21–8.

[69] Pengzhan Y, Ning L, Xiguang L, Gefei Z, Quanbin Z, Pengcheng L. Antihyperlipidemic effects of different molecular weight sulfated polysaccharides from *Ulva pertusa* (Chlorophyta). Pharmacol Res. 2003;48(6):543–9.

[70] Qi H, Zhang Q, Zhao T, Chen R, Zhang H, Niu X, . Antioxidant activity of different sulfate content derivatives of polysaccharide extracted from *Ulva pertusa* (Chlorophyta) in vitro. Int J Biol Macromol. 2005;37(4):195–9.

[71] Pengzhan Y, Quanbin Z, Ning L, Zuhong X, Yanmei W, Zhi'en L. Polysaccharides from *Ulva pertusa* (Chlorophyta) and preliminary studies on their antihyperlipidemia activity. J Appl Phycol. 2003;15(1):21–7.

[72] Bobin-Dubigeon C, Lahaye M, Barry J-L. Human colonic bacterial degradability of dietary fibres from sea-lettuce (*Ulva* sp.). J Sci Food Agric. 1997;73(2):149–59.

[73] Fernández PV, Ciancia M, Miravalles AB, Estevez JM. Cell-wall polymer mapping in the coenocytic macroalga *Codium vermilara* (Bryopsidales, Chlorophyta)1. J Phycol. 2010;46(3):456–65.

[74] Estevez JM, Fernández PV, Kasulin L, Dupree P, Ciancia M. Chemical and in situ characterization of macromolecular components of the cell walls from the green seaweed *Codium fragile*. Glycobiology. 2009;19(3):212–28.

[75] Zhang Z, Wang F, Wang X, Liu X, Hou Y, Zhang Q. Extraction of the polysaccharides from five algae and their potential antioxidant activity in vitro. Carbohydr Polym. 2010;82(1):118–21.

[76] Blomster J, Maggs CA, Stanhope MJ. Molecular and morphological analysis of *Enteromorpha intestinalis* and *E. Compressa* (Chlorophyta) in the British Isles. J Phycol. 1998;34(2):319–40.

[77] Jiao G, Yu G, Wang W, Zhao X, Zhang J, Ewart SH. Properties of polysaccharides in several seaweeds from Atlantic Canada and their potential anti-influenza viral activities. J Ocean Univ China. 2012;11(2):205–12.

[78] Santos SAO, Vilela C, Freire CSR, Abreu MH, Rocha SM, Silvestre AJD. Chlorophyta and Rhodophyta macroalgae: A source of health promoting phytochemicals. Food Chem. 2015;183:122–8.

[79] Celikler S, Tas S, Vatan O, Ziyanok-Ayvalik S, Yildiz G, Bilaloglu R. Anti-hyperglycemic and antigenotoxic potential of *Ulva rigida* ethanolic extract in the experimental diabetes mellitus. Food Chem Toxicol Int J Publ Br Ind Biol Res Assoc. 2009;47(8):1837–40.

[80] Bocanegra A, Bastida S, Benedí J, Nus M, Sánchez-Montero JM, Sánchez-Muniz FJ. Effect of seaweed and cholesterol-enriched diets on postprandial lipoproteinaemia in rats. Br J Nutr. 2009;102(12):1728–39.

[81] Qi H, Liu X, Zhang J, Duan Y, Wang X, Zhang Q. Synthesis and antihyperlipidemic activity of acetylated derivative of Ulvan from *Ulva pertusa*. Int J Biol Macromol. 2012;50(1):270–2.

[82] Yangthong M, Hutadilok-Towatana N, Phromkunthong W. Antioxidant activities of four edible seaweeds from the southern coast of Thailand. Plant Foods Hum Nutr Dordr Neth. 2009;64(3):218–23.

[83] Farasat M, Khavari-Nejad R-A, Nabavi SMB, Namjooyan F. Antioxidant activity, total phenolics and flavonoid contents of some edible green seaweeds from northern coasts of the Persian Gulf. Iran J Pharm Res IJPR. 2014;13(1):163–70.

Section 2

Alternative Cropping Systems

Chapter 3

Traditional Raised-Floor Granary and Rice Production Cycle in Bali: Past, Present, and Future of Balinese Agriculture

Leo Aoi Hosoya

Additional information is available at the end of the chapter

http://dx.doi.org/10.5772/62643

Abstract

A granary can represent a certain set of farming activities reflecting cultural and regional characteristics, and also be associated with symbolic meanings. The traditional raised-floor rice granary in Bali, Indonesia, called a *Lumbung*, only survives in specific areas of the island today. What is the factor underlying its survival and disappearance? The results of the author's field research in Bali from 2006 to 2011 indicate that this is connected with the survival of local rice production, which was Bali's traditional rice before being overtaken by the highly productive normal rice—introduced in the 1960s and 1970s. Today, local rice is cultivated only in a few specific areas such as Tabanan prefecture, where not only *Lumbung*s but also a set of traditional farming customs are still used. In addition, a clear conceptual connection between *Lumbung*s and local rice is observed, Such that local rice is exclusively offered in a *Lumbung* to the goddess Dewi Suri. Such practices suggest that the introduction and spread of the new normal rice not only changed the type of rice cultivated but also led to the decrease of traditional or "real" farming practices among local farmers, as represented by the decline of the *Lumbung*.

Keywords: Granary, Crop production cycle, Cultural identity, Agricultural landscape, Paddy rice farming, Ethnohistory

1. Introduction: *Lumbung* (raised-floor granary) and rice production cycle in Bali

This chapter discusses the *Lumbung*, a Balinese traditional raised-floor rice granary, and its relationship with the production cycle of rice and local farmers' perceptions of it. The author uses ethnohistorical research and proposes a measure for the proper preservation of the *Lumbung* as a symbol for the promotion of agriculture in the future.

Architecture is the materialization of the function of a human activity space and thus represents certain set of human activities reflecting cultural and regional characteristics. Therefore, traditional architecture can be associated with not only practical activities but also symbolic meanings including the concept of sacredness and taboo and cultural identity. In the preservation of traditional architecture, we must therefore take a holistic view of both the practical and symbolic aspects of traditional structures in the mental landscape of local populations.

Among the various types of architecture, granaries are among the most commonly seen constructions. Food storage facilities emerged in the very early stages of human history and played a fundamental role in everyday landscapes [1]. The style of a granary not only reflects the subsistence strategy of each society but also the characteristics of its culture. Granaries have also been symbolic objects or stages for ceremonies and thus concern the human mental landscape.

Many ethnographic researchers have become interested in traditional granaries and their past functions and symbolism. For example, in Japanese scholarship, research has been mainly conducted in subtropical islands, such as [2–5] Amami and Okinawa Islands, Japan. These studies noted that sacredness or display of political power or wealth is associated with traditional granaries. Accordingly, a granary could be an instrument for connecting the economical and daily act of storing food with sacredness and politics. On the other hand, the perspectives of those studies tended to be limited to granaries themselves; the relationships of granaries to the overall routine associated with subsistence have not been sufficiently discussed. This ethnographic study on Bali focuses on this aspect of traditional granaries.

Bali has a traditional raised-floor granary for rice. Previously, granaries were called by several names depending on their size, as will be explained below. However, the number of granaries remaining today is much smaller, and size distinctions have been lost; therefore, in this chapter, traditional Balinese granaries are referred to as *Lumbung*s, which is now the most commonly used term in modern Bali.

Rice farming is vital in Balinese culture, and the *Lumbung* has played a significant role in Balinese life; however, the tradition now only survives in limited places. Here, the author would like to discuss the role of the *Lumbung* in the Balinese rice production cycle and the factors underlying its survival and gradual disappearance, using data obtained from field work carried out from 2006 to 2011. The *Lumbung* can be an important cultural symbol for Bali and useful for reviving agricultural practices. Thus, understanding local people's perceptions of the *Lumbung* is important for the future planning of the Balinese agricultural landscape.

2. Background of the research: the history of *Lumbung*

Bali is a province of Indonesia and is located to the east of Java. It has a population of 3.89 million (as of 2010), covering 5633 km^2 (**Figure 1**). Because of its location near the equator, its

http://dx.doi.org/10.5772/62643

year-round temperatures range between 23 and 31°C, and the average annual rainfall is around 2000 mm in the province capital, Denpasar. It has a tropical humid climate with a dry season from April to November and a wet season from December to March [6–8]. The island is divided into eight prefectures (*Kabupaten*) inheriting the regional divisions from the Klungkung dynasty and the seven small kingdoms from the seventeenth to eighteenth centuries [6]. 93.18% of its population is Hindu and referred to as "Balinese Hindu" [6], and the *Bali Aga* and *Bali Mula* communities comprise the minorities [6]. The author's ethnographical studies target the Balinese Hindu population.

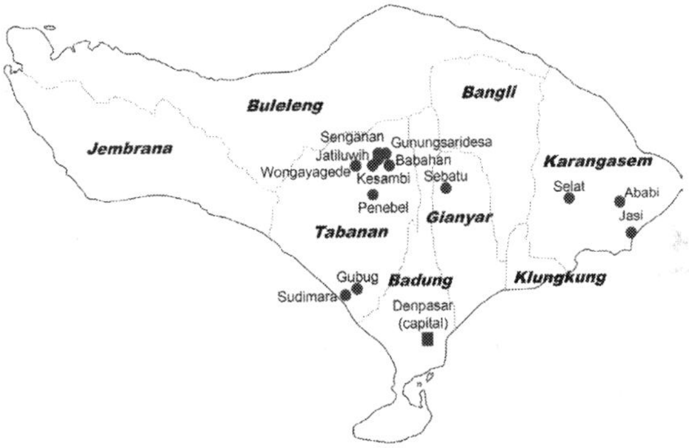

Figure 1. The map of Bali and locations of field research areas.

The *Lumbung*, the theme of this research, is a Balinese traditional raised-floor rice granary with a gable roof. Today, such granaries are only used in a few specific areas, mainly in Tabanan prefecture; however, a few decades ago, they were common sights in the Balinese agricultural landscape.

Covarrubias [9], a Mexican painter who lived in Bali in the 1930s, documented various aspects of the contemporary Balinese culture. Among them, he mentioned the raised-floor granary, noting that it was called by different names according to its size, such as *Lumbung, Glebeg, Djineng, Kelumpu*, and *Kelingkin*, in order of importance. According to Covarrubias, "a granary symbolized the economic status of a family," and the structure is "similar to a yam house in Melanesia" with a thatched gable roof and four pillars attached with rat guards [9: pp. 107] (translated by Hosoya). He also recorded certain taboos associated with granaries, such as that against speaking while bringing out rice in the daytime and the condition that a person entering a granary be mentally and physically healthy and not chew betel nuts. Covarrubias's description suggests that granaries were a common part of the Balinese landscape.

This standing of granaries in Bali appears to have continued into the 1960s. The book edited by Miyamoto [10], conducted as part of the "Rice Farming Culture in Southeast Asia" project, is a good authority on Bali during this period, with rather detailed descriptions of granaries as a part of rice farming culture. Ishikawa [11], as a member of the same project, recorded the classifications for granaries in Sesetan village, south of the capital city Denpasar. According to him, granaries that stocked more than 800 rice sheaves (10–11 kg/bundle) were called *Keling*, those holding more than 200 sheaves were called *Djineng*, and those holding more than 100 sheaves were called *Kelumpu*. Ishikawa also described the granaries as having gable roofs thatched with *Alang-alang/lalang* (a kind of reed) grass and noted that some granaries had an additional floor beneath the raised floor for a workshop space, which was sometimes surrounded by a bamboo mat that served as a wall. There were also several rules regarding these granaries; for instance, they were always constructed near the kitchen in the southern part of a house complex, and when there were two wives in a household, they could have separate kitchens but had to share one granary. It is also reported cases in Pantjur village in Lombok Island, an island east of the main Bali Island, where granaries were also classified by the size: The larger ones were the *Lumbung*, and smaller ones were the *Sambi*. In case of the *Lumbung*, an additional floor was built beneath the raised floor as a workshop space [11]. When one household had both the larger and smaller granaries, the two may be connected by an extended roof, and the in-between space could be used as a cowshed. These records in [11] show that granaries in the 1960s were still a common part of the Balinese landscape and also a fundamental part of daily life.

However, in 1980s, it appears that the situation started to change, namely *Lumbung* seems to have become out of use except a particular region. In Kagami's discussion [12] of the contemporary Bali house complex, he observed that "… today, more and more families process and sell rice directly from the field, and [traditional] granaries are falling out of use even if a family owns one" (translated by Hosoya). On the other hand, Nagafuchi [13] observed that the *Mantenin* ceremony for raised-floor granaries was still regularly practiced in the Wongayagede village, Tabanan prefecture, indicating regular use of granaries. These studies show that by the late 1980s, the raised-floor granary had become a disappearing tradition except in the specific area of Tabanan prefecture, where it continued being a part of the everyday landscape and was still actively used. This 1980s pattern is basically what can be observed today, and Tabanan prefecture is the main area of *Lumbung* survival.

These records on raised-floor granaries in Bali indicated that a remarkable shift occurred in the use and popularity of granaries in the 1970s and 1980s. What was the change? Why did the raised-floor granary disappear in most areas in Bali, and why did it survive in specific areas such as Tabanan prefecture? To answer these questions, the study of the present state of the *Lumbung* and its cultural background, with a comparative view of the areas where it has survived and disappeared, would be useful. This will also provide a clue to understanding the significance of the *Lumbung* in the Balinese agricultural landscape today. To this end, the author carried out a field research in Balinese farming villages.

3. Field research (2006–2011)

The field research was conducted from 2006 to 2011, and the detailed results have been published elsewhere [1, 14–18]. The research method involved interviewing farming families on the *Lumbung* and observing agricultural activities/ceremonies concerning the *Lumbung*. The interviewees were mainly comprised of *Lumbung* owners in Tabanan, Gianyar, and Karangasem prefectures, but for comparative study, farmers without *Lumbungs* in Karangasem prefecture were also interviewed. Detailed information on the interviewees is shown in **Table 1**. Names of the interviewees are given as initials to protect their privacy. The spellings of village names are based on those in the "Bali Street Atlas, 2005/2006 edition" (Periplus Editions).

Prefecture (*Kabupaten*)	Village (*Desa*)	Informants			Cultivated rice	No. of *Lumbung*
Tabanan	Babahan	BB1	Men (75 and 40 years old)	Land owner	Local 1*/year, normal 1/year, *Keten*	1
	Gunungsaridesa	GN1	Man (62 years old); Woman (53 years old)	Land owner	Local 1–2/year, normal 2/year, *Keten*	14
		GN2	Man (86 years old)	Land owner	Local 1–2/year, normal 1/year, *Injin, Keten*	1
	Jati Luwih	JT1	Woman (38 years old)	Land owner	Local 1/year, normal 1/year, *Injin, Keten*	3
		JT2	Woman (30s?)	Land owner	Local 1/year, normal 1/year, Injin, Keten	2
		JT3	Woman (60 years old)	Land owner	Local 1/year, normal 1/year	5
		JT4	Man (27 years old)	Land owner	Local 1/year, normal 1/year	4
	Kesambi	KS1	Woman (55 years old)	Land owner	Local 2/year, normal 1/year	1
	Penebel	PN1	Woman (75 years old); Man (46 years old)	Land owner**	Local 1/year, normal 1/year	1
	Senganan	SG1	Man (80 years old)	Land owner	Local 1/year, normal 1/year	1
		SG2	Men (42 years old & 36 years old)	Land owner	Local 1/Year, normal 2/year, *Keten*	3
	Wongayagede	WG1	Man (45 years old)	Land owner	Local 2/year, *Injin* 2/year	1

Prefecture (*Kabupaten*)	Village (*Desa*)	Informants			Cultivated rice	No. of *Lumbung*
		WG2	Woman (60s?)	Land owner	Local, *Injin*	2
	Gubug	GB1	Woman (80 years old)	Land owner	Normal 3/year	2
		GB2	Woman (60s?)	Land owner	Normal 2/year	1
	Sudimara	SD1	Man (55 years old)	Land owner	Normal 2/year	2
Gianyar	Sebatu	SB1	Man (45 years old)	land owner	Local 2/year, *Injin, Keten*	3
Karangasem	Ababi	AB1	Woman (65 years old)	Land owner**	Normal 2–3/year	1
	Jasi	JS1	Man (50 years old)	Land owner	Normal 3/year	none
		JS2	Woman (50s?)	Tenant	Normal	none
		JS3	Man (64 years old)	Tenant	Normal	none
	Selat	SL1	Man (60 years old)	Tenant	Local 1/year, normal 2/year. *Injin, Keten*	none
		SL2	Man (70 years old)	Land owner	Local, normal, *Injin, Keten*	none (1 *Tukub*)
		SL3	Woman (43 years old)	Land owner	Normal 2/year, *Keten*	1

*The number indicates harvest number within 1 year shifting.
**Not farming his/herself.

Table 1. Backgrounds of informants.

3.1. Survival of the *Lumbung* and its relationship to rice type

The results of the field research suggested the high possibility that the survival of the *Lumbung* is strongly tied to the type of rice cultivated. Here, I introduce the present status of the *Lumbung* as observed through the fieldwork and then demonstrate that its relationship with cultivated rice is the key to explaining why *Lumbung*s have survived in specific areas of modern Bali while disappearing in other areas.

http://dx.doi.org/10.5772/62643

3.1.1. *Lumbung* today

As previously mentioned, the author interviewed primarily households that owned *Lumbungs*, with a few exceptions for comparative purposes. Accordingly, the research area was limited to Tabanan, Gianyar, and Karangasem prefectures. It must be noted that in other areas, namely the majority of Bali farming lands, *Lumbungs* no longer exist.

The surviving *Lumbungs* observed by the author have either four or six posts but exhibit no notable differences in size corresponding to those recorded in historical documents such as [9, 11]. However, interviewee GN1 explained that *Lumbungs* with six posts were built when abundant rice harvests were expected and paddy fields were large, so the difference in the number of posts may be a relic of the diversity of the *Lumbung* sizes.

The *Lumbung* roof was traditionally thatched by *Alang-alang* grass, as described by [9, 11], and some old *Lumbungs* still retain this traditional style of roofing (**Figure 2**). However, over the last several decades, almost all farmers have chosen metal roofs to replace thatched ones when rebuilding roofs (**Figure 3**), mainly because of the cost: While a thatched roof costs 3–5 million rupia, a metal roof costs only 0.8 million rupia (GB1, SD1, in the interview in 2007). It is also difficult today to find *Alang-alang* grass or to employ workers capable of thatching. At the same time, many interviewees cited the advantages of metal roofs over thatched ones, such as more durability (JT3, GN1), more effective for keeping off rats (JT3, SB1), and better for drying stored rice (SB1). Metal roofs therefore appear to be a positive introduction.

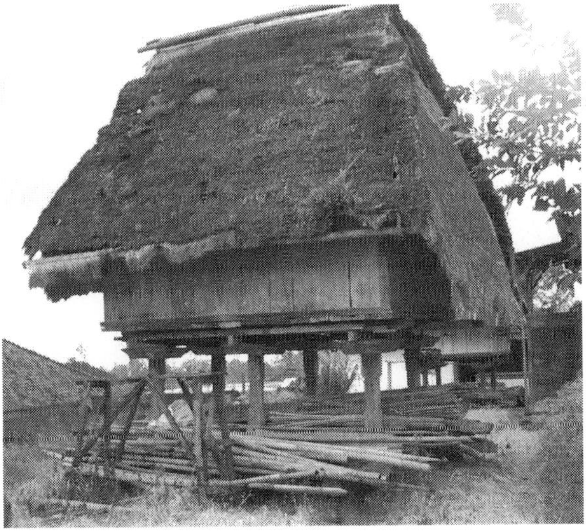

Figure 2. Traditional style of *Lumbung*.

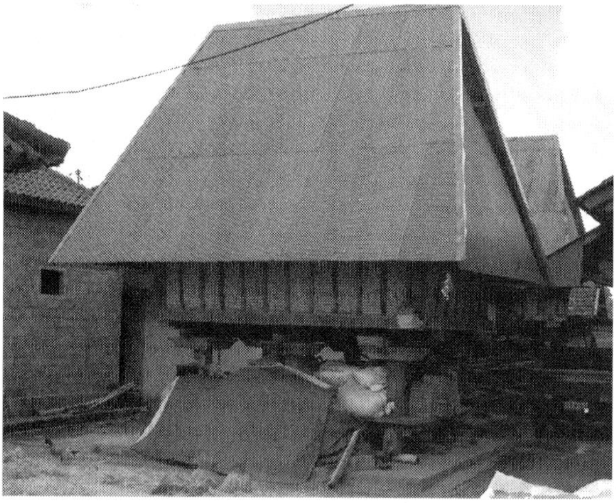

Figure 3. *Lumbung* with a metal roof.

Most *Lumbungs* have a second floor beneath the raised floor (**Figure 4**), as reported in [11] in 1960s. The second floor is used for various purposes (as an eating space, a resting space, a meeting space with a guest, and so on), but many interviewees (PN1, GB1, SD1, SL3, GN1, etc.) said that it was used for preparation for *Lumbung*-related ceremonies. Indeed, the author observed this ceremonial usage and was also often invited into the space for interviews or dining.

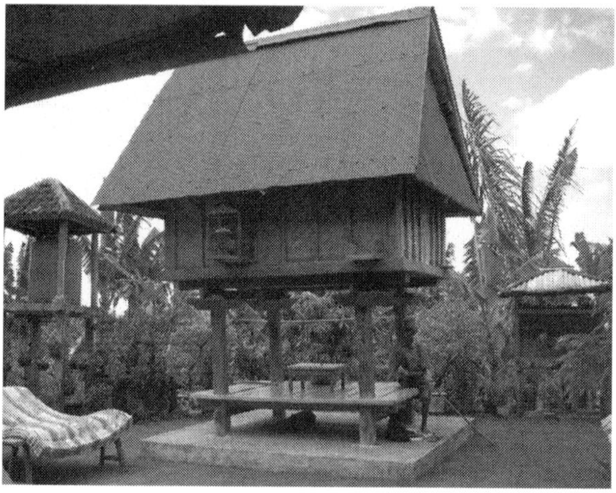

Figure 4. Utilization of the second floor beneath the raised-floor of a *Lumbung*.

http://dx.doi.org/10.5772/62643

Some *Lumbungs*, in particular, the ones that have rather recently been renovated, are decorated, sometimes quite elaborately, with carvings and coloring (**Figure 5**) (eg., PN1 renovated 16 years ago; GN2, 3 months ago; BB2, 2 years ago). Decoration, the means of which vary, is normally done by a family member, but it also can be done by an architect (BB1). According to GN2, the purpose of decoration is "showing off."

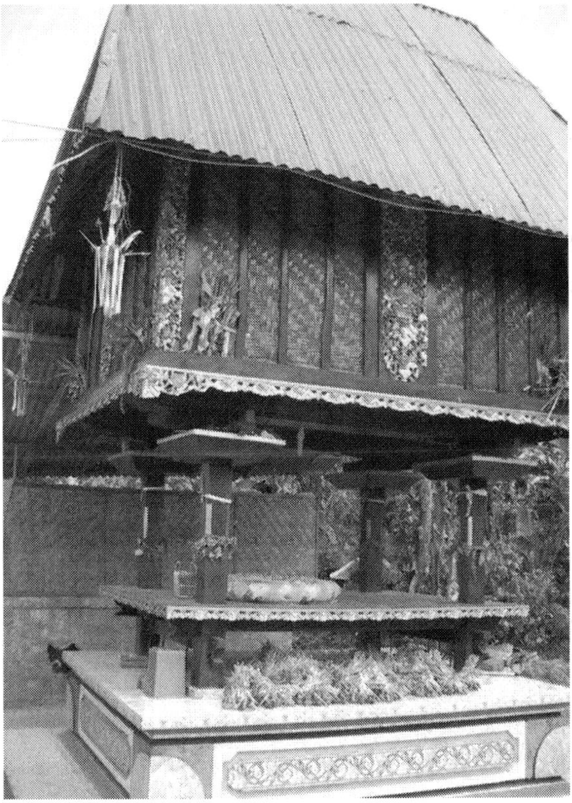

Figure 5. Decorated *Lumbung*.

In Wongayagede village, Tabanan prefecture, the shape of *Lumbungs* is quite characteristic. *Lumbungs* observed by the author in this village and the nearby Tengkudak and Penatahan villages were uniformly bell-shaped with a red tile roof (**Figure 6**). In Tengkudak village, there was a metal-roofed *Lumbung*, which was also bell-shaped. The author could not determine the origin of this specific *Lumbung* shape despite interviewing several farmers, but the shape resembles that of typical Balinese temples, suggesting some possible connection. It is reported [13, 19] that Wongayagede village was a special village in a religious context, as village residents were in charge of managing ceremonies at Luhur Batukau Temple located in the north of the village, at the foot of Batukau Mountain. In the village, *Injin,* black rice specially used to make ceremonial cakes, was also intensively produced [15].

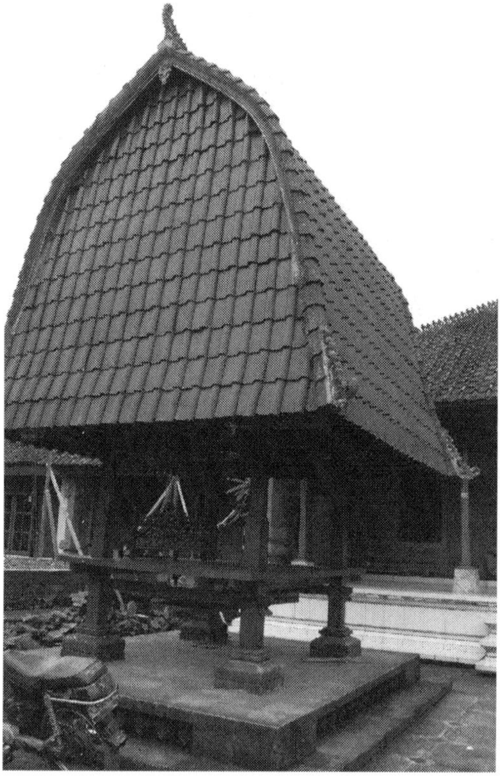

Figure 6. *Lumbung* of Wangayagede village.

Several regulations and taboos associated with *Lumbung*s were recorded in [9, 11], as was shown in Section 2, but many of them are now obsolete.

It is reported in [11] that the *Lumbung* had to be in the south part relative to the house complex. Some farmers mentioned that today, it must be constructed in the south (PN1, JT2, and JT3) or in the south or west (KS1). However, many farmers claim, "It can be constructed anywhere there is space" (GB1, SD1, JT4, SG1, SG2, AB1). Therefore, this condition seems to be gradually losing importance. Indeed, BB1 reported, "Once, it had to be in the south, but it doesn't matter now." Some interviewees also said that the door of a *Lumbung* must face south or west (JT3, JT4, SG2, AB1).

http://dx.doi.org/10.5772/62643

None of the *Lumbung*-related taboos recorded by Covarrubias [9] were mentioned by the interviewees. Instead, most of them mentioned the same two taboos: "Women on their period cannot enter a *Lumbung*" and "Rice cannot be taken out from a *Lumbung* on particular days." These "particular days" varied by interviewee, such as specific days of a week, a day of a ceremony, or the day of the new moon/full moon. Other taboos mentioned by interviewees were as follows: "Rice cannot be taken out repeatedly on the same day, and no one can look inside the *Lumbung* on a day rice is taken out" (GN2), and "Anyone can put rice into a *Lumbung*, but only the owner couple can take rice out; even a child of the couple cannot do that" (JT2). Other interviewees denied the existence of any taboo (PN1, AB1).

In terms of the symbolism associated with the *Lumbung*, normally, some rice sheaves placed in the *Lumbung* are carefully separated from the rice for consumption by placing them on a beam, in a basket, or else, as an offering for Dewi Sri, the goddess of rice. In some cases, the offering rice is replaced regularly with new rice, but in others, it stays unchanged for several decades. The detail is explained in the next section, as it is connected with the issue of the rice types. Furthermore, a ceremony for rice harvest and storage called *Mantenin* is still regularly held in particular areas, mainly in Tabanan prefecture. Although the original concept of *Mantenin* seems to be a celebration of rice granaries in general, it seems to be rather exclusively associated with the *Lumbung*. This notion is also explained below.

3.1.2. The *Lumbung* and cultivated rice

Next, we discuss how the type of cultivated rice and the survival of *Lumbung* are related according to the field research results.

Paddy field rice cultivation was introduced in Bali through the Dong Son culture, which spread across Southeast Asia around the fifth to third centuries BC [7]. Paddy field rice became the staple food of the islanders, and paddy fields were reported to occupy 17% of the island's area in the 1960s [20]. Today, rice is still the fundamental food in Bali, and a meal is not considered "proper" without rice [15]. Tubers, which are eaten as staple foods in many other tropical regions, and bread, which was introduced through Western cultures, are also eaten but are treated as merely snacks. Rice is also considered the best of all crops [6]. In the author's interview, many interviewees said that "rice is the food of human beings, but tubers are for pigs" (such as JT1, JT3, WG1, SD1, JS1, JS2 SL2, SL3).

In present-day Bali, two types of rice are cultivated. One is the traditional "local rice (*Padi Bali*)" in red and white variations, and the other is the more recently introduced normal rice (*Beras*)." Along with these, the black rice *Injin* and red and white *Ketan* varieties for making ceremonial cakes are also cultivated (for detail, see [14]). Normal rice was introduced as a part of the BIMAS (*Bimbingan Massal* = group instruction) and IMMAS (*Intensifikasi Massal* = group intensification) Programs promoted by the Indonesian government in 1960s and 1970s [21]. Today, normal rice production is prevalent in Bali because of its higher yields than local rice and is promoted by the government, but in certain areas, local rice continues to be regularly cultivated. In present-day Bali, rice can normally be harvested 2–3 times a year, and in many cases, local rice farmers cultivate both local rice and normal rice in rotation within 1 year (see **Table 1**). Yet, some farmers still only cultivate local rice.

Tabanan prefecture is a representative and well-known area of local rice farming, and most of these also cultivate normal rice. Among the author's interviewees, only the farmers of Wongayagede village cultivated local rice but not normal rice. In addition, the field research revealed villages in other prefectures that also regularly cultivated local rice, namely Sabato village in Gianyar prefecture and Selat and Ababi villages in Karangasem prefecture. In case of the villages in Karangasem, only specific households of the villages continued exclusive local rice cultivation. Among these, a household in Sabato and one in Selat cultivated local rice only, but other households produced local rice and normal rice.

In general, those regions of continued local rice cultivation seem to originally have had high yields of rice because of rich water sources. On the other hand, the areas that have now completely turned to normal rice cultivation seem to have had lower rice production. Before the introduction of normal rice, the current yields of 2–3 rice harvests per year were impossible except in especially productive areas such as Tabanan prefecture. In other areas, farmers rotated cultivation of rice and dry field crops such as tubers and peanuts. It is recorded in [20] that in the 1960s, rotating cultivation was practiced in 70% of Bali's farmlands. According to the author's interviews with farmers, local rice cultivation is still maintained in the few areas where multiple rice harvests were possible even before the introduction of normal rice introduction, whereas in the rotating-cultivation areas, which comprise the majority of Balinese farmlands, the introduction of normal rice now enables several rice harvests a year. In these areas, rotating cultivation with dry field crops is still conducted as needed.

The author's field research surveyed 24 households (**Table 1**), and among them, 19 owned *Lumbungs*. The 19 households can be categorized into three groups by their rice cultivation patterns: (1) cultivating local rice only; (2) cultivating local rice and normal rice alternately within one year; and (3) cultivating normal rice only. Among these groups, there seem to be characteristic differences in the ways the *Lumbungs* are used. These provide a clue to understanding the significance of the *Lumbung* in Balinese farming.

Three households in Wongayagede of Tabanan and Sebatu of Gianyar (WB1, WB2, SB1) fit into category 1. Remarkably, their *Lumbungs* were extremely well-maintained with frequent reconstructions positively introducing new material for better rice storage, such as tiled roofs and concrete walls, as well as new decorative designs. In SB1's case, it is notable that a new *Lumbung,* in addition to an existing two, was created only 15 years ago, which rarely occurs today. The interviewee said that the new *Lumbung* was needed: "Because we have too much rice production, two *Lumbungs* were not enough to store it." The older two *Lumbangs* were passed on to their first son, whereas the new one was given to their second son. Formerly, Balinese custom dictated that when a son became independent and had his own family, he received a new granary even if he continued living in his old household with its own raised-floor granary [11]. However, today, the custom seems to have almost disappeared because of the shrinking number of *Lumbungs*, and new ones are rarely constructed. However, in the case of SB1, the old custom was still followed in part.

http://dx.doi.org/10.5772/62643

The majority of the surveyed households (11) fit into category 2 and were all in Tabanan prefecture. The noticeable feature of *Lumbung* usage in these households was that although they cultivated both local and normal rice within one year in most cases, the *Lumbungs* were used exclusively to store local rice. Normal rice was stored elsewhere, such as in the main residence or in a storage shed without a raised-floor or not constructed in the traditional style. KS1 from the Kesambi village was the exception and stored both types of rice in the *Lumbung*, explaining "We have only a small paddy field, and the rice production is not very high, so we store everything in the *Lumbung*" (KS1). The most common explanation for the different storage spaces for different types of rice was the difference in harvesting methods: Local rice is picked the head, which are bundled into sheaves for storage (**Figure 7**), whereas normal rice is cut at the bottom of the stalks and threshed in the field (**Figure 8,9**), with the grains stored in sacks. Normal rice sacks are generally heavy (20–30 kg) and difficult to carry up a raised-floor *Lumbung*, which could be one reason why only local rice is stored in the *Lumbungs*. However, this cannot explain why both types of storage are maintained despite the high maintenance costs of *Lumbungs*, rather than storing both local and normal rice in new sheds. This raises the possibility of a perceptual connection between the *Lumbung* and local rice, rather than a logistical necessity.

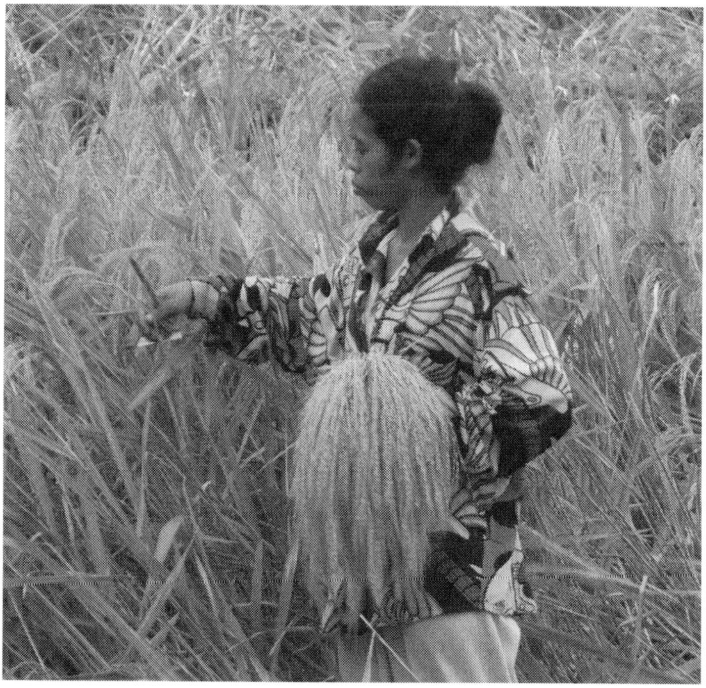

Figure 7. Harvesting local rice.

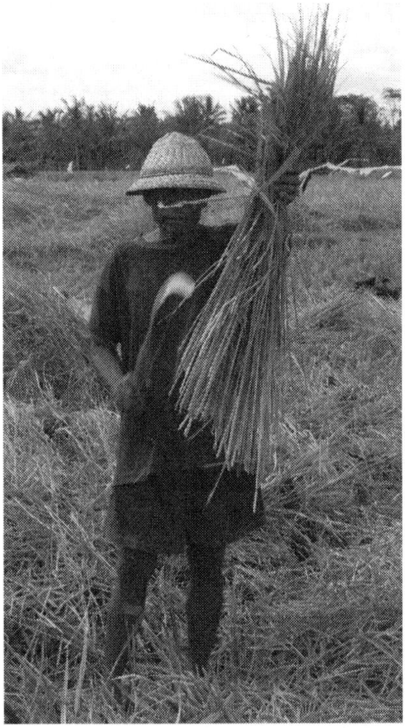

Figure 8. Harvesting normal rice.

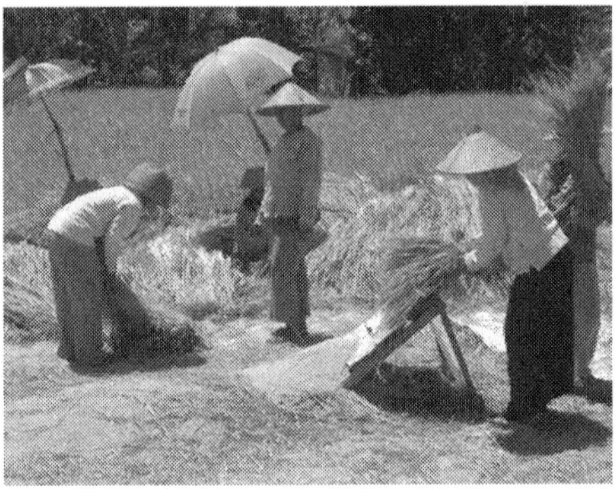

Figure 9. Normal rice threshing in the field.

Five households fall into category 3, that is, only cultivating normal rice. Of these, three were in the South Tabanan villages of Gubug and Sudimara, and one each was in the villages of Ababi and Selat in Karangasem. In fact, these were rather exceptional cases since the majority of farmers in Bali who cultivate only normal rice do not own *Lumbungs*. In these cases of category 3, the *Lumbungs* were generally old and poorly maintained. In the case of SL3 in Selat village, the *Lumbung* was not used at all. In the author's 2008 interview, SL3 said "When we switched to normal rice 10 years ago, we stopped storing new harvests in the *Lumbung*. Then, 3 years ago, we used up all the remaining local rice storage in the *Lumbung*, and it has been empty since then. But we keep it because it was passed down from our ancestors, so we do not dare destroy it." However, when the author made a second visit in 2011, SL3's *Lumbung* had been replaced by a small shop (*Warun*) run by the family. In other cases of category 3, *Lumbungs* were still used for storing normal rice, but this use did not appear to be out of necessity. Some interviewees provided explanations: "Because I got it from my mother, I maintain it" (AB1) and "As a *Lumbung* is precious, I will use it until it breaks" (SD1). These responses indicate that *Lumbungs* are relics for them to maintain for the sake of tradition rather than daily use. This conceptual shift regarding the *Lumbung* seems to have occurred when normal rice was introduced, as most obviously evident in the case of SL3. The cases in category 3 again show the conceptual connection between local rice and the *Lumbung*.

For the comparative study, the author also interviewed some households without *Lumbung* in Karangasem prefecture. In the case of SL2 of Selat village, the household cultivated both local and normal rice in a year, and they stored local rice in a storage facility called a *Tukub*, which is another traditional facility with a bamboo-thatched roof, an attic to store rice in, and a ground floor for storing other objects. SL2 had owned it for more than 65 years. The family used to own a *Lumbung* as well, but it was demolished with the introduction of normal rice cultivation in 1970s. In three cases from Jasi village (JS1, JS2, and JS3), the interviewees were exclusively normal rice farmers and had no memories of the *Lumbung*.

In summary, these examples show that the *Lumbung* is evidently connected with local rice cultivation and plays an active role only in local rice production areas. According to the author's research, all households still cultivating traditional local rice own a *Lumbung* (categories 1 and 2), and these *Lumbungs* are not just maintained but actively used, with regular maintenance and refurbishing. Some *Lumbungs* are even elaborately decorated or remodeled with new materials and structures. In households cultivating only local rice (category 1), *Lumbungs* are used the most intensively, and even new ones are being constructed. Farmers cultivating both local rice and normal rice (category 2) commonly store only local rice in *Lumbungs*, whereas normal rice is stored elsewhere, which demonstrates an obvious connection between the *Lumbung* and local rice. In contrast, in category 3, that is, those no longer cultivating local rice, *Lumbungs* seem to be treated as relics or mementos rather than essential parts of the agricultural routine; consequently, maintenance or refurbishment is rarely performed.

Therefore, the survival of the *Lumbung* seems closely related to the survival of local rice production. This view is reasonable from a historical perspective as well as the introduction of normal rice in the 1970s and 1980s coincides with the gradual decline in the popularity of the *Lumbung*.

Next, we discuss the fundamental difference between local rice and normal rice production routines and their connection to the *Lumbung*.

3.2. Comparison of production routines of local rice and normal rice

It has already been mentioned that the harvesting methods of local rice and normal rice clearly differed, and other conspicuous differences also distinguished their production and processing routines.

First, the tools used in their production were typically different. The most obvious difference was in the harvesting tools. To harvest local rice, a traditional handmade picker called an *Anggapan* (**Figure 10**) was used. It is a tool with a hand-sized wooden body and an attached metal edge. Their shapes varied as they were made by the farmers themselves. In contrast, mass-produced sickles (*Arit*) were used for normal rice harvest. Thus, traditional tools and the production techniques were exclusively related to local rice. In addition, local rice was threshed and dehusked with a traditional mortar (large mortar: *Katungan*, small mortar: *Lesung*) and pestle (*Luu*) until 30–40 years ago (according to interviews with PN1, SL1, BB1, KS1, SB1, SL2). Stored local rice sheaves were brought out part by part for several days' use and threshed and dehusked near a *Lumbung*. However, this work has now been almost completely replaced by mechanical threshing and dehusking by a machine owned by the village. The shift to this method occurred 30–40 years ago, at the same time as the introduction of normal rice, and indeed, some interviewees concurred that machine threshing and dehusking were introduced with normal rice (SL2, AB1).

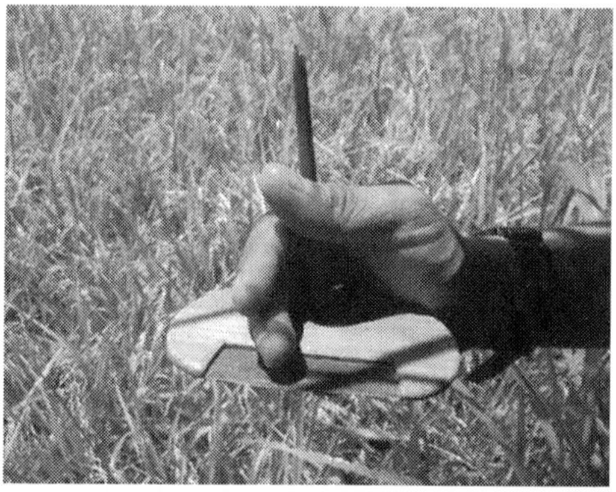

Figure 10. Traditional handmade picker (*Anggapan*) for local rice.

Second, the organization of planting and harvesting also differed between the two rice types. On the one hand, both planting and harvesting of local rice were basically conducted on a family basis, and normally, fewer than five people worked together in the field. Sometimes, other farmers from the village joined to help in keeping with the traditional *Gotong Royong* system, in which farmers in a village help each other, and the reward is not money but tea/ snacks and a share of the harvested rice (see also [19]). Even in these cases, however, the work is still done on a small scale. On the other hand, planting and harvesting of normal rice were done by a group of tenants led by a landlord, and harvesting, in particular, was done on a large scale. Normal rice was threshed immediately after the harvest in the field, and the threshed grains were packed into sacks, so around 10 people normally worked together for this. However, the households farming both local rice and normal rice (those typically found in Tabanan prefecture) used the same harvesting method for normal rice (harvesting and threshing conducted in sequence in the field), but this work was still done on a family basis on a small scale. This shows that the difference in work organization between local rice and normal rice is not a mere reflection of different harvesting methods but rather a conceptual divide: Local rice farmers today apply the family-based working style to the introduced normal rice as well.

In connection with the work organization issue, the rhythm of annual work scheduling also seems to differ between local rice and normal rice farmers. Local rice farmers plant and harvest rice on a fixed schedule shared with other farmers in their village, whereas normal rice planting and harvesting are rather random in timing, even within in a single village (for details, see [15]). In addition, several ceremonies were traditionally performed at critical stages of the rice production cycle by the whole village [15]. While these ceremonies are mostly no longer observed, the village-shared scheduling of farming routines again seems to reflect a more traditional way of farming.

In addition, the gender division in work responsibilities appeared to differ between the two types of rice, though information collected in this study on this area is still limited. Interviewee BB1 said "Rice harvesting has been the responsibility of women from the old times. But anyone can harvest normal rice." Indeed, normal rice was normally harvested by a mixed group of men and women, according to the author's observation, whereas almost all harvesting workers for local rice were women. Furthermore, all interviewees said that threshing and dehusking with a mortar and a pestle were exclusively women's job, but this work division was discontinued when the threshing and dehusking machine was introduced. It is suggested that traditional gender roles could have also disappeared with the introduction of normal rice and new farming techniques.

Third, the author also conducted interviews regarding the farmers' perceptions of the two rice types, and, again, clear differences emerged. When asked about local rice, all the interviewees gave positive comments such as "I love the taste" (JT1, JT3, SG1), "It contains a lot of vitamins" (SG2, SB1, KS1), "It is filling" (JT3), "It is not easily infected by germs" (AB1, JT3), and "It does not require much fertilizer" (AB1). It is intriguing that even AB1, who had already completely stopped producing local rice, made such comments. In contrast, the only positive, uniform comment all interviewees made about normal rice was "It can be harvested more quickly than local rice." Obviously, local rice holds special value for Balinese farmers that normal rice does not despite the fact that normal rice production is now much more common across Bali.

Apparently reflecting this perception, many farmers who cultivate both local and normal rice (such as JT1, JT3, BB1, SL2, GN2) clearly distinguished the uses of the two types of rice: Local rice was for home consumption, and normal rice was for selling outside the community. In fact, the standard price of local rice in the market was higher than that of normal rice. According to the interviewees the author interviewed in July 2006, local rice sold at 6000–7000 rupia per kilogram, whereas normal rice sold for 4500 rupia per kilogram. Therefore, for profit, it would be better to sell local rice and eat normal rice themselves, but in reality, farmers do the opposite. This also shows the strong mental attachment to local rice among Balinese farmers. Yet, it must be also noted that some people who were not originally farmers but started farming as a business have recently begun cultivating local rice to sell for profit (such as PN1). This suggests that the perceptions of Balinese rice farming are gradually shifting.

Related to the perception issue, ritual practices related to rice farming also seemed to be influenced by the introduction of normal rice. Bali is called the "Island of the Gods" because of the numerous ceremonies and offerings for various occasions, which are deeply rooted in Balinese daily life. There are also a number of ceremonies associated with rice farming (see [15]), though some of these, particularly village-based ceremonies, are no longer regularly practiced, as mentioned above. *Mantenin*, the ceremony for rice granaries after a new harvest, is one of the farming ceremonies still practiced with certain regularity but only in households with a traditional *Lumbung*. Furthermore, these ceremonies are observed differently among such households, depending on the types of rice they cultivate. Basically, when a family cultivates local rice, they regularly hold *Mantenin*. Even in the case of SL2, who cultivated local rice but replaced the household's *Lumbung* with another traditional storage facility (a *Tukub*), *Mantenin* was observed, albeit on a small scale. In cases of families cultivating both local and normal rice, while *Mantenin* was observed for harvests of both types of rice, the scale of the ceremony was smaller with normal rice (JT1, GN1). In households that owned *Lumbung*s but no longer cultivated local rice, the situation varied. SD1 reported using both a *Lumbung* and a modern storehouse for normal rice and observing *Mantenin* for both storage facilities. However, the ceremony was much simpler with the modern storehouse, as the author directly observed. GB1 reported a similar situation of using a *Lumbung* for normal rice, but they had stopped holding *Mantenin*. Instead, they conducted a ceremony for the goddess Dewi Sri, who is believed to reside in the *Lumbung*, twice a year regardless of the actual harvest timings. Furthermore, in the case of SL3, who owned a *Lumbung* but did not use it, they stopped holding *Mantenin* at the same time they stopped cultivating local rice. This suggests that the regular and proper observance of *Mantenin* depended on the presence of local rice production rather than that of a *Lumbung* itself. It is noted in [6] that Balinese people did not practice farming ceremonies for cash crops despite their deeply rooted tradition of farming ceremonies. The simplified *Mantenin* for normal rice may reflect the local perception of normal rice as more like a cash crop than a subsistence one.

In addition, it is notable that the rice placed in a *Lumbung* as an offering for Dewi Suri was exclusively local rice, even when normal rice was stored in the *Lumbung*. Among those the author interviewed about the offering rice, WG1, BB1, JT1, and SB1 were local rice producers who stored only local rice in *Lumbung*s. In their cases, not only was local rice the offering but

http://dx.doi.org/10.5772/62643

also the offering activities seemed comparatively frequent. WB1 headed a household that cultivated local rice only, and they offered fresh rice from every harvest, or every 6 months. BB1, JT1, and SB1 grew both local and normal rice but stored only the former in a *Lumbung*. BB1 reported adding fresh rice little by little to the existing offering rice during every local rice harvest. The rice added was picked just before starting the harvest. When the amount of the offering rice become too large, the whole offering rice pile was removed from the *Lumbung* and burnt, and the ash was scattered in the paddy field. In JT1's *Lumbung*, approximately 1 kg of local rice was placed as an offering, and although the rice was not regularly replaced, it was regularly removed for the annual *Mesabe* ceremony offered at a temple and returned to the *Lumbung* after the ceremony. In SB1's *Lumbung*, five or six sheaves of local rice were placed as an offering and kept there for a "long time" (SB1) but regularly taken out as offerings for various ceremonies.

KS1 was also a local and normal rice producer and, in contrast to other such farmers, stored both types of rice together in the *Lumbung*, as mentioned above. However, although both types of rice were stored in the *Lumbung*, rice for offerings in the *Lumbung* exclusively had to be local rice. The offering rice was replaced over a period of several years.

SD1 did not produce local rice at all and stored normal rice in the *Lumbung*. Nevertheless, SD1's offering rice in the *Lumbung* was local rice, though quite an old stock. They stopped cultivating local rice in 1965, but following the will of the interviewee's father, who had died "30 years ago" (SD1), a basket of local rice was kept in the *Lumbung* as an offering "till it crumbles away" (SD1). Again, the offering rice in these different cases showed that the custom is still a part of daily life for local rice farmers but only a traditional relic for normal rice farmers.

Above all, it can be said that the introduction of normal rice not only resulted in the shift in the type of cultivated rice but also led to the erosion of traditional farming routines, tool making, work organization, gender-based labor divisions, and ritual practices. On the basis of these field research results, we now discuss the reasons for the disappearance/survival of the *Lumbung* and their meaning.

4. Discussion: what is the significance of the *Lumbung*?

The preceding discussion raises the question of the nature of connection between the *Lumbung* and local rice. The authors' field research revealed that the routine of local rice production was significantly different from that of normal rice production. Local rice was harvested by a handmade tool, the *Anggapan*, and the sheaf was dried and stored in a *Lumbung*. The work was generally done on a family basis. On the other hand, normal rice was harvested by a mass-produced *Arit*, and the grains put into sacks and stored in a non-traditional storehouse. Because normal rice harvesting and threshing were carried out together, related labor tended to be on a larger scale and commonly involved a large group of tenant farmers. In addition, traditional gender-based divisions of labor and mutual supporting systems in communities were more visible in the local rice production area. Differences between the two types of rice were also reflected in the rituals surrounding rice storage. Specifically, traditional ceremonies and taboos were retained with the *Lumbung* but were not observed with normal rice storage facilities.

In summary, it appears that agricultural activities associated with local and normal rice form coherent circles (**Figure 11**). All elements involved in local rice production, such as working style, utilities, and tools used, seem to be based on tradition. On the other hand, activities for normal rice production seem to be based on the concept of efficiency, positively introducing new styles of work. It is thus likely that the *Lumbung* can find a reason to exist as a part of the traditional cycle of local rice but cannot accommodate the efficiency circle of normal rice. This explains why *Lumbungs* started to disappear at the same time local rice cultivation disappeared, while their active use in local rice cultivation continues.

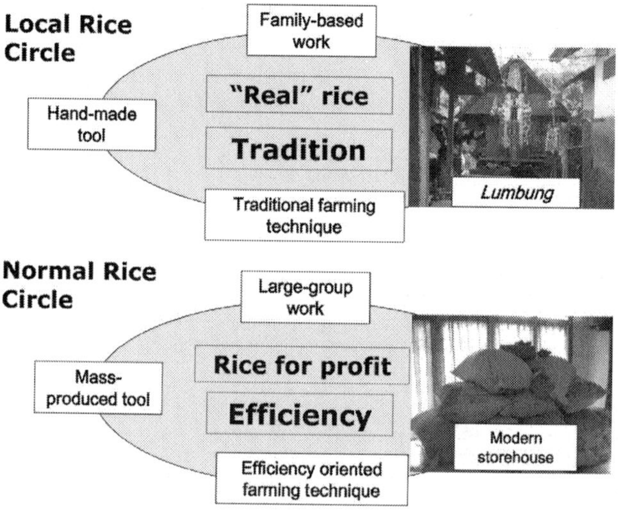

Figure 11. Conceptual circles concerning local rice and normal rice.

Moreover, it seems that each of the two coherent circles is sustained by different shifts in the mentality of Balinese people. In interviews, farmers often expressed a strong mental attachment to local rice, even those who no longer cultivated it, describing it as "tasty," "good," "nutritious," and so on. Almost all the farmers said that they would like to eat local rice as much as possible. In contrast, no value was attached to normal rice other than its being "productive." Indeed, among farmers mix-cultivating local and normal rice, many said that they saved local rice for their own consumption and sold normal rice commercially. This reflects the perception of local rice as real food and normal rice as more of a cash crop. The general consensus was that because local rice is real food, it is produced in a more "real" way using traditional facilities and tools and proper ceremonies, whereas with people do not care about normal rice and thus change their production methods for greater efficiency.

http://dx.doi.org/10.5772/62643

Above all, the traditional circle of local rice seems to be sustained by the Balinese people's idea of "real rice production," and the *Lumbung*, which is the most visible factor in the circle in the everyday landscape, symbolizes the idea. Therefore, if *Lumbung*s are properly protected and presented in the planning of the Balinese landscape, it can be usefully connected to the protection of Balinese farming culture and people's motivation to farm.

5. Prospects: promotion of agriculture in Bali and the *Lumbung*

In modern-day Bali, the decrease of farmlands and populations under the pressure of the tourism industry is a serious problem. To promote rice farming, it would be effective to protect local rice cultivation and *Lumbung*s as part of the whole agricultural landscape and to encourage local people to work with these to affirm their own cultural identity.

Although rice terraces in Tabanan and Gianyar are among the most popular and highly promoted sightseeing spots, *Lumbung*s, which are an indispensable factor in traditional rice farming, are not sufficiently promoted or protected. Traditional and characteristic styles of store houses also exist in other parts of the world, such as the yam house in Papua New Guinea and the *Takakura* raised-floor granary in the Amami Oshima Island, Japan [18, 22]. Because of their distinctive shapes, these store houses are heavily promoted as symbols of local culture (e.g., the miniature models are sold as souvenirs, and the models are displayed in important places such as airports of the Amami Oshima Island, the Papua New Guinean Diet Building, and sightseeing spots of those areas). On the other hand, Bali's *Lumbung*s are not as well promoted. At present, they are treated as cultural icons only in limited areas, such as the *Lumbung* display at some souvenir shops around Ubud and a new *Lumbung*-shaped hotel by the Bali Nature Land in Gunungsaridesa, Tabanan. It will be useful to promote the *Lumbung* as a Balinese cultural symbol more broadly because it can contribute much to those who consider agricultural work their own cultural identity and promote agriculture along with tourism.

Acknowledgements

The field research was supported by the Grants-in-Aid of Ministry of Education, Culture, Sports, Science and Technology (MEXT) below: Promotion Grant "Constructing Foundation for Japanese Archaeobotany: Data collection of Jomon and Yayoi excavated botanical remains and ethnographic research" (No. 17904030, Fiscal Year 2005, Principal Investigator: Aoi Hosoya), Grant-in-Aid (A) "Ritual and Landscape of Paddy Rice Culture in East Asian Villages" (Fiscal Year 2004–2007, Principal Investigator: Tadashi Ebisawa), and Young Scientists Starting-up Grant "Rethinking Prehistoric Subsistence Strategy in Japan Archipelago: Ethnographic research to construct foundation of archaeobotany" (No. 19820059, Fiscal Year 2007–2008, Principal Investigator: Aoi Hosoya)

The author would also like to thank Professor Takuma Yogo (Waseda University) for his great help for the author to start research in Bali, Mr Nyoman Lai for his thorough work as a translator and driver, and Enago (www.enago.jp) for the English language review.

Author details

Leo Aoi Hosoya

Ochanomizu University, Tokyo, Japan

References

[1] Hosoya A. Rice granary: the landmark of paddy rice culture. In: Uchiyama J, Lindstrom K, editors. Landscape History and Environment on the East Asian Inland Seas 1: Versatile Waterfronts" Part II. Showado Publications: Kyoto; 2010. pp. 49–73 (in Japanese).

[2] Sakai U. Raised-floor granary and ceremony space. Bulletin of the Folklore Society of Japan. 1974; 93: 14–27 (in Japanese).

[3] Kurumizawa K. Group granaries. Material Culture. 1987; 48: 78–83 (in Japanese).

[4] Asakawa S. Ethnoarchaeology of raised-floor granaries. In: Naoki K, Ogasawara Y, editors. Granaries and Ancient Kingships. Minerva Shobo: Kyoto; 1991 (in Japanese).

[5] Muratake S. The Structure of Ceremonial Spaces: Social Anthropology Reports. Tokyo University Press: Tokyo; 1984. 239 p (in Japanese).

[6] Yoshida T. Balinese: The Cosmology of Ceremonies and Flowers. Kobundo: Tokyo; 1992. 196 p (in Japanese).

[7] Yoshihara Y. Overview of the Bali Island. In: Yoshida T, editor. Bali, the Island of Gods: Ceremonies and Entertainments of Bali Hindu. Shunju Sha: Tokyo; 1994. pp. 13–29 (in Japanese).

[8] Kijima M. Bali rice terrace, protected by gods and people. Consultant. 2006; 230: 38–41 (in Japanese).

[9] Covarrubias M. Island of Bali. Alfred A. Knopf, Inc.: New York; 1936 (translated into Japanese by Sekimoto K. Heibon Sha: Tokyo; 1991. 418 p.).

[10] Miyamoto N, editor. Studies of the Bali Islanders: Synthetic Research of the Culture of Rice-cultivating Races in Southeast Asian Countries (II). Tokai University Press: Kanagawa; 1968. 222 p (in Japanese).

[11] Ishikawa E. Farmers families and the living style in Bali and Lonbok Islands. In: Miyamoto N, editor. Studies of the Bali Islanders: Synthetic Research of the Culture of Rice-

cultivating Races in Southeast Asian Countries (II). Tokai University Press: Kanagawa; 1968. pp. 1–59 (in Japanese).

[12] Kagami H. Living in Harmony with the Cosmos. Ethnology Quarterly. 1987; 42: 63–71 (in Japanese).

[13] Nagafuchi Y. The World of Offering: Mantenin Padi ceremony in Wongayagede, Bali. Ethnology Quarterly. 1988; 45: 32–41 (in Japanese).

[14] Hosoya A. Ethnographic Research on Rice Farming in Bali from a Viewpoint of 'Social Archaeobotany'. Journal of Southeast Asian Archaeology. 2007; 27: 19–38 (in Japanese).

[15] Hosoya A. Rice and granary: ethnographic research of Bali paddy rice agriculture. In: Ebisawa T, editor. Study of Paddy Rice Culture IV: Bali Paddy Rice Agriculture and Ceremonies. Waseda University Institute of Paddy Field Culture: Tokyo; 2008. pp. 87–111 (in Japanese).

[16] Hosoya A. Storage system and living cycle: ethnographic research of Bali paddy rice agriculture and Papua New Guinean swidden agriculture. In: Japanese Archaeological Association 2008 Aichi Meeting Organization Committee, editor. Proceedings of Japanese Archaeological Association 2008 Aichi Meeting. Nanzan University: Aichi; 2008. pp. 309–324 (in Japanese).

[17] Hosoya A. Significance of storage facility: comparative ethnoarchaeology of Bali and Papua New Guinea. In: Kikuchi T, editor. New Horizon of Comparative Archaeology. Dosei Sha: Tokyo; 2010. pp. 742–752 (in Japanese).

[18] Hosoya LA. Surviving tradition and disappearing tradition: 'Old Days' landscape with raised-floor granaries in Bali and Amami Oshima Islands. In: Kinda A, Komeie T, Minamide S, Mizoguchi T, Uesugi K, editors. Proceedings of the 14th International Conference of Historical Geographers Kyoto 2009. Kyoto University Press: Kyoto; 2010. pp. 218–219.

[19] Nagafuchi Y. Bali, Religion, Nation: Tracing Institutionalization of Hindu. Seido Sha: Tokyo; 2007. 311 p (in Japanese).

[20] Fujioka Y. Bali paddy rice cultivation and the related ceremonies. In: Miyamoto N, editor. Studies of the Bali Islanders: Synthetic Research of the Culture of Rice-cultivating Races in Southeast Asian Countries (II). Tokai University Press: Kanagawa; 1968. pp. 95–151 (in Japanese).

[21] Murai Y, Saeki N. Indonesia - After Suharto. Iwanami Shoten: Tokyo; 1998. 61 p (in Japanese)

[22] Hosoya A. The swidden farming cycle and storage system of tuber crops: Papua New Guinean case studies and diversity of farming society. In: Sato YI, Kimura E, editors. The History of Eurasian Agriculture 4: Various Cultivars and Farming Culture. Rinsen shoten: Kyoto; 2009. pp. 185–228 (in Japanese).

Chapter 4

Potential of Improving Agronomic Attributes in Tropical Legumes Using Two Mutation Breeding Techniques in Southern Africa

E. T. Gwata, H. Shimelis and P. M. Matova

Additional information is available at the end of the chapter

http://dx.doi.org/10.5772/62262

Abstract

Tropical legumes such as cowpea (*Vigna unguiculata*) and tepary bean (*Phaseolus acutifolius*) are important in traditional smallholder cropping systems, particularly in sub-Saharan Africa. Both legumes are adapted to harsh environments including extreme temperatures, drought and poor soil fertility. They provide affordable sources of protein for human consumption and are valuable for income generation. These crops contribute significantly to soil fertility improvement through biological nitrogen fixation. In many parts of Africa, the productivity of these legumes is generally low partly because farmers grow unimproved varieties that are often produced for subsistence purposes on poor soils in mixed cropping systems with limited production inputs. Therefore, this research was designed to evaluate the potential of two distinct mutation breeding approaches in creating useful genetic variation in the two legumes in order to improve the agronomic attributes of both crops. The variation was determined by measuring a range of agronomic traits at both the seedling and adult plant stages. The results showed significant genetic variation among cowpea mutants that were induced with various doses of gamma radiation as well as among tepary bean mutants that were induced with a chemical mutagenic agent, ethyl methanesulphonate (EMS). The optimum doses at LD_{50} for two cowpea genotypes (Nakare and Shindimba) were ≤200 Gy while the third genotype (Bira) tolerated a dose three-fold higher. In the EMS mutagenesis of tepary bean, the estimated LD_{50} was ≤2.4% EMS (v/v). In both approaches, percent seed germination decreased with increased dose and the coefficients of determination for the linear functions were high (>75%), suggesting that there were notable associations between the reduction in seed germination and the concentration of the mutagen. At the adult plant stage, tepary bean showed that the mutant generation significantly ($P < 0.05$) influenced positively the important agronomic traits such as shoot dry weight, number of pods per branch and seed size. Dose effects were also significant for seed size. The field trials conducted in Zimbabwe showed >10.0% increase in both seed size and grain yield potential of some mutant cowpea genotypes compared with the standard check. These findings provide reference doses for large-scale gamma irradiation of cowpea as well as chemical mutagenesis for tepary bean. In addition, the germplasm produced from these approaches has the potential for selection in a range of agro-ecological conditions across the region, thus creating alternative cropping systems for the smallholder growers.

Keywords: cowpea, genotype, legumes, mutagenesis, tepary bean

1. Introduction

Tropical legumes such as cowpea (*Vigna unguiculata*) and tepary bean (*Phaseolus acutifolius*) are important in traditional smallholder cropping systems, particularly in sub-Saharan Africa. Both legumes are adapted to harsh environments including extreme temperatures, drought and poor soil fertility [1–3]. Cowpea was domesticated in Southern Africa where its wild relatives are found [4] and it is cultivated widely in many countries in the region including Namibia, South Africa and Zimbabwe. In contrast, tepary bean is indigenous to the south-western parts of the United States and Mexico [5], but spread to many African countries including Botswana, Kenya, Malawi, South Africa and Zimbabwe where smallholder farmers use unimproved landraces of the crop. The grain of both cowpea and tepary bean provide affordable sources of protein for human consumption and are valuable for income generation, particularly in the smallholder cropping systems in southern Africa. In addition, the legumes contribute significantly to soil fertility improvement through biological nitrogen fixation [6,7] and are often produced in intercrops with maize (*Zea mays*), sorghum (*Sorghum bicolor*) and millets (*Pennisetum* spp.) that are popular in the region.

Despite these important uses, the productivity of these legumes is generally low (<500.0 kg/ha), partly because farmers grow unimproved varieties which are often produced for subsistence purposes on poor soils in mixed cropping systems with limited production inputs. In addition, the genetic base of each of these legumes is narrow, particularly for exploiting important economic traits such as grain yield and tolerance to insect pests. However, mutation breeding has the potential to generate unique genetic variations in crops that can be exploited by plant breeders in the development of new cultivars [8]. The success of mutation breeding has been reported widely in legumes [9–13], cereals [14,15] and several other crops such as sunflower [16], cassava [17] and oilseed rape [18]. In mutation breeding, artificial mutagenesis is induced on crop germplasm using various types of mutagenic agents such as gamma rays or ethyl methanesulphonate (EMS) followed by selection of useful traits from the resulting mutants. The approach has the potential to produce desirable results faster than conventional plant breeding methods [19]. In this chapter, we present research work which was designed to evaluate the potential of two distinct mutation breeding approaches in creating useful genetic variation in cowpea and tepary bean in order to improve the agronomic attributes of both crops. The development of improved cultivars of these legumes using diverse germplasm from southern Africa will benefit breeding programs as well as growers and end-users in the region.

2. Materials and methods

The study consisted of three components involving separate artificial mutagenesis of batches of cowpea seeds and tepary bean, followed by evaluation of seedlings under greenhouse or laboratory conditions. In addition, the agronomic field performance of both cowpea and tepary bean mutants was conducted. The field evaluation of cowpea mutant lines utilized distinct agro-ecological conditions in Zimbabwe (**Table 1**). The early generations of tepary bean mutants were evaluated at a representative location in the semi-arid region of northern South Africa.

Test location	Co-ordinates	Soil type	Annual rainfall (mm)	Summer temperatures (°C)
Thohoyandou (South Africa)	22°58'S; 30°26'E	Red well- drained, clay	500 to 920	22–40
Gwebi Variety Testing Centre (Zimbabwe)	17°41'S 30°32'E	Red clay	700–1000	17–30
Save Valley Research Station (Zimbabwe)	21°02'S 31°57'E	Alluvial	<450	15–37
Matopos Research Station (Zimbabwe)	20°24'S 28°28'E	Black clays	450–650	15–29

Table 1. The characteristics of the test locations used in the study.

2.1. Cowpea genetic material and its mutagenesis

In the first part of the study, batches of about 150 seeds (in three replications) of each of three cowpea genotypes (Nakare, Shindimba and Bira) were gamma-irradiated at the facility at the International Atomic Energy Agency (IAEA), Agriculture and Biotechnology Laboratory (Austria) using a range of irradiation doses (0, 100, 200, 300, 400, 500 and 600 Gy) [20] in order to determine the optimum irradiation level causing optimum mutation frequency and subsequently planted in a greenhouse. Similarly, the M_1 seed of one cowpea genotype (CBC-1, originating from Zimbabwe), which was gamma-irradiated at the same facility in Austria, was planted in the greenhouse initially in order to raise M_2 plants. Subsequent successive generations (from which several experimental lines were isolated) were raised at the Crop Breeding Institute (Harare, Zimbabwe).

2.1.1. Seedling evaluation and measurements

The mutagenized seeds (M_1) were planted in a greenhouse at the IAEA (Austria) in seedling trays with a medium consisting of peat, sand and vermiculate at a ratio of 2:1:1, respectively. The temperature and photoperiod in the greenhouse were maintained at 28.0°C and 12.0 h, respectively. The soil moisture was maintained by watering twice per week. A completely randomized experimental design with three replications was used for the study. The percent germination (%G) was measured 7 days after planting, but the epicotyl and hypocotyl lengths were measured 14 days after planting. The measurements that were obtained for the %G were used for determining the LD_{50} for each genotype which was estimated with the aid of a linear regression model using a simple straight line equation $y = mx + c$ [where: y = the response variable (%G), x = the independent variable (irradiation dose); m = the slope and c = the constant].

2.1.2. *Field evaluation and measurements*

Fourteen M_6 cowpea mutant genotypes together with two standard checks were evaluated in the field at three distinct locations in Zimbabwe (**Table 1**). The seed of each genotype was planted in two-row field plots spaced at 0.45 m apart × 0.15 m intra-row spacing and arranged in a randomized complete block design replicated four times. Standard cowpea management practices were followed at Gwebi Variety Testing Centre (G.V.T.C.) and Matopos Research Station (M.R.S.). The field trial at Save Valley Research Station (S.V.R.S.) was conducted during the off-season period in winter under irrigation. The location experiences no frost in winter.

At each location, six agronomic traits were measured as follows:

(i) duration to 50.0% flowering (50%DF) (ii) duration to 95.0% maturity (95%DM) (iii) number of pods per plant (NPP) (iv) number of seeds per pod (NSP) (v) 100 seed weight (100-SW) and (vi) grain yield (GY).

2.2. Tepary bean genetic material and its mutagenesis

Three genotypes of tepary bean (GEN-1; GEN-4; GEN-6) that were obtained originally from growers in Sekhukhune District (Limpopo Province, South Africa) were used in the study. These genotypes were self-fertilized for five cycles in order to maximize homozygosity prior to chemical mutagenesis. The selfing was conducted in the greenhouse at the University of Venda (Thohoyandou, South Africa). The seed mutagenesis was conducted at the University of KwaZulu Natal (Pietermaritzburg, South Africa). A sample of healthy clean seeds (approximately 250) of each genotype was surface-sterilized by soaking in 70% ethanol for 1 min and rinsing three times followed by soaking in 30% sodium hypochlorite bleach solution (2% NaOCl) for 10 min before rinsing again three times in tap water. The seed was then soaked in distilled water for 12 h at room temperature. Each seed sample was partitioned into smaller batches (containing about 50 seeds each) and placed in specially designed sachets made of nylon mesh (measuring about 7.0 cm in width × 11.0 cm in length) [21]. The seed was transferred to aqueous solutions of varying doses (0.0, 0.5, 1.0, 1.5, 2.0 v/v) of EMS and incubated at room temperature for 1 h after which the treated seed was rinsed under running tap water for 2 h in order to remove the excess EMS and enable safe handling. A portion of the M_1 seed (75%) was used for evaluating the seedling traits while the remainder was planted in the greenhouse in order to raise the M_2 to M_4 seed for the subsequent field evaluation.

2.2.1. Seedling evaluation and measurements

The mutagenized seed samples (M_1) were germinated in plastic jars (7.5 cm diameter × 8.0 cm height, lined with moist filter paper at the base) in the laboratory at room temperature. At the first initiation of the first trifoliate leaf, several seedling traits were measured including (i) percent seed germination (%G), (ii) number of secondary roots (NSR), (iii) primary root length (PRL) (mm), (iv) secondary root length (SRL) (mm) and (v) shoot height (mm) (SHT).

2.2.2. Field evaluation and measurements

The seed of each treatment combination (generation × genotype × dose) was planted separately (in plots spaced at 0.1 m within the row and 0.6 m between the rows) in the field under rain-fed conditions. A three-factorial arrangement laid out in a randomized complete block design was used in the study. At the reproductive stage or maturity, a range of agronomic attributes were measured including the (i) number of primary branches per plant (NPB) (ii) pod length (PL) (iii) shoot dry weight (SDW) (iv) 100 seed weight (100-SW).

3. Results and discussion

3.1. Seedling performance of cowpea mutants

A significant ($P < 0.01$) interaction occurred between cowpea genotypes and gamma radiation doses, suggesting that there were differential responses to the irradiation doses among the cultivars. The %G decreased drastically with increased irradiation dose in all the three cultivars. At 600.0 Gy, seed germination (47.9%) occurred only in cultivar 'Bira'. The highest LD_{50} (689.00 Gy) was observed for cultivar 'Bira' (**Table 2**), which suggested that this cultivar was the most resistant to gamma radiation.

Cowpea cultivar	Linear equation	LD_{50} (Gy)
Nakare	$y = -0.17x + 78.09$	165.24
Shindimba	$y = -0.16x + 81.79$	198.69
Bira	$y = -0.08x + 105.12$	689.00

Table 2. The LD_{50} of three cowpea cultivars that were irradiated with gamma rays in order to induce mutation.

Radiation doses >200.0 Gy significantly reduced the epicotyl and hypocotyl lengths in both 'Nakare' and 'Shindimba', but at 0.0 Gy the longest epicotyl (3.11 cm) and hypocotyl (6.71 cm) were observed in the cultivar 'Nakare' [20]. In general, both the epicotyl and the hypocotyl lengths decreased as the gamma irradiation doses increased. Between 400.0 and 600.0 Gy, the hypocotyl growth occurred only in cultivar 'Bira'.

The coefficient of determination (R^2) estimated from the linear regression equations for both traits were high (ranging from 76.0–93.0%), suggesting that there was a notable association between the reduction of epicotyl and hypocotyl lengths due to increased radiation doses. These results showed genotypic variation in tolerance to gamma radiation with 'Bira' tolerating the heaviest doses of radiation. Therefore, from a crop improvement standpoint, it is critical to determine the optimum dose of irradiation for each candidate cowpea genotype prior to large-scale blanket mutagenesis with the gamma radiation approach. Ideally, the irradiation doses for generating useful mutants in crop improvement programs should be within ±5 units of the experimentally determined optimal dose [17]. Nonetheless, induced mutations are random events such that, in all probability, their reproducibility in each candidate genotype with the same mutagen is highly unlikely.

3.2. Agronomic field performance of cowpea mutants

During the advancement of the mutagenized generations, the cowpea mutants derived from 'CBC-1' using gamma radiation revealed two notable phenotypes namely earliness (**Figure 1**) and above canopy pod development (**Figure 2**). Early maturity is particularly important as a mechanism for escaping drought. There were significant ($P < 0.05$) differences only in the duration to 50.0% flowering (50%DF) and grain yield (GY) over the three consecutive cropping seasons (starting from 2012/2013) at G.V.T.C. in Zimbabwe. This indicated that, to all intents and purposes, the majority of the useful agronomic traits of the mutants were stable after the M_5 generation. At the location, the highest grain yield (0.87 t/ha) was attained by the mutant line 'CM/250/M6-6'. In all the selected elite lines, the desirable traits were induced by using a relatively low-range (150.0–250.0 Gy) dose of gamma radiation in the original parental line (CBC-1).

The results also showed that there was no significant variability for the duration to 95.0% maturity (95%DM) or the number of pods per plant (NPP) or the number of seeds per pod (NSP), suggesting that the selected elite lines were uniform with regard to these traits. However, the mean NPP (9.0) was considerably lower in comparison with observations from other studies [22]. In a similar study that evaluated cowpea M_1 genotypes, the NPP was reduced from 43 to 17 by exposure to 400.0 Gy [9]. However, the mean NSP was consistent with other findings [23].

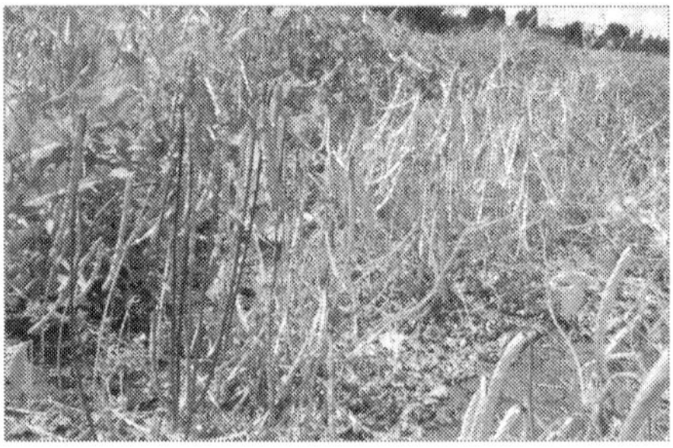

Figure 1. Some cowpea mutant lines showed early maturity.

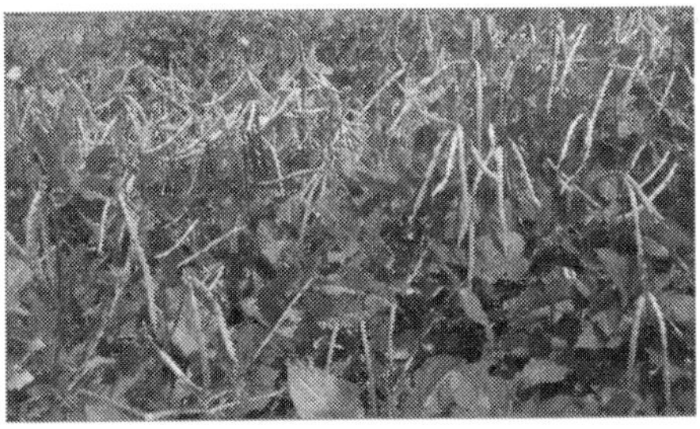

Figure 2. Cowpea pods developed above the canopy in some mutant lines.

Mutant line	50%DF	95%DM	NPP	NSP	100-SW (g)	GY (t/ha)
CM/200/M6-2	60.00 a	95.66 a	21.33 a	15.33 a	14.33 abc	1.19 a
CBC-2	59.00 a	95.66 a	21.33 a	15.00 a	12.67 c	1.43 a
CM/250/M6-5	59.00 a	95.33 a	22.33 a	15.33 a	15.67 a	1.57 a
CM/250/M6-2	59.67 a	97.33 a	23.00 a	14.00 a	13.33 bc	1.21 a
CM/150/M6-1	60.67 a	97.33 a	28.00 a	15.00 a	15.67 a	1.72 a
CM/200/M6-3	60.67 a	95.33 a	22.33 a	14.00 a	15.67 a	1.15 a
CM/250/M6-1	59.67 a	95.67 a	21.67 a	13.67 a	15.00 ab	1.21 a
CM/250/M6-7	58.00 a	94.33 a	14.33 a	14.00 a	15.00 ab	1.28 a
CM/250/M6-4	60.67 a	94.33 a	22.67 a	15.00 a	15.00 ab	1.24 a
CBC-1	61.00 a	95.33 a	21.33 a	15.67 a	15.00 ab	1.29 a
CM/150/M6-3	60.33 a	96.33 a	18.33 a	14.33 a	14.33 abc	1.16 a
CM/200/M6-4	58.00 a	95.00 a	21.67 a	14.00 a	13.67 abc	1.38 a
CM/150/M6-2	59.33 a	94.33 a	18.33 a	13.33 a	15.33 ab	1.32 a
CM/200/M6-1	58.67 a	95.00 a	23.00 a	15.00 a	14.33 abc	1.41 a
CM/250/M6-6	61.00 a	94.67 a	18.00 a	13.33 a	14.33 abc	1.36 a
CM/250/M6-3	60.00 a	95.67 a	19.00 a	14.33 a	15.00 ab	1.21 a
Mean	59.73	95.46	21.02	14.46	14.64	1.32
C.V.	2.24	1.47	22.08	8.71	7.90	23.85
Significance	NS	NS	NS	NS	*	NS

Means followed by the same letter in each column are not significantly different ($P < 0.05$).
NS = not significant at the 5.0% probability level; * = not significant at the 5.0% probability level.
[50%DF = duration to 50% flowering; 95%DM = duration to 95% maturity; NPP = number of pods per plant; NSP = number of seeds per pod; 100-SW = 100 seed weight; GY = grain yield].

Table 3. Mean performance of cowpea M_6 experimental lines over two cropping seasons at the Matopos Research Station (Zimbabwe).

At M.R.S., the highest yield was attained by the experimental cultivar 'CM/150/M6-1' (**Table 3**). The average NPP (21.0) increased by more than two-fold (**Table 4**) while both the 50%DF and the 95%DM increased markedly in comparison with the other two locations, suggesting that the agro-ecological conditions were more favourable at this location than at G.V.T.C. for this sample of cowpea experimental lines. This trend was more apparent when the germplasm was evaluated during winter but under irrigation at the S.V.R.S. where all the genotypes attained >4.0 t/ha grain yield (**Figure 3**). The line 'CM/150/M6-1' achieved the highest (6.36 t/ha) which represented almost 20.0% grain yield advantage over the check cultivar. In addition, four genotypes achieved >10.0% higher grain yield over the check cultivar 'CBC-2' (**Figure 4**). These results demonstrated the potential of the newly developed genotypes to increase the productivity of cowpea significantly particularly under favourable conditions such as those at S.V.R.S.

Test location	50%DF (d)	95%DM (d)	NPP	NSP	100-SW (g)	GY (t/ha)
Gwebi Variety Testing Centre	53.50	78.78	9.00	11.78	13.91	0.75
Matopos Research Station	59.73	95.46	21.02	14.46	14.64	1.32
Save Valley Research Station	86.63	129.25	19.06	12.13	14.19	5.49

Table 4. Mean performance of cowpea M_6 experimental lines at three locations in Zimbabwe.

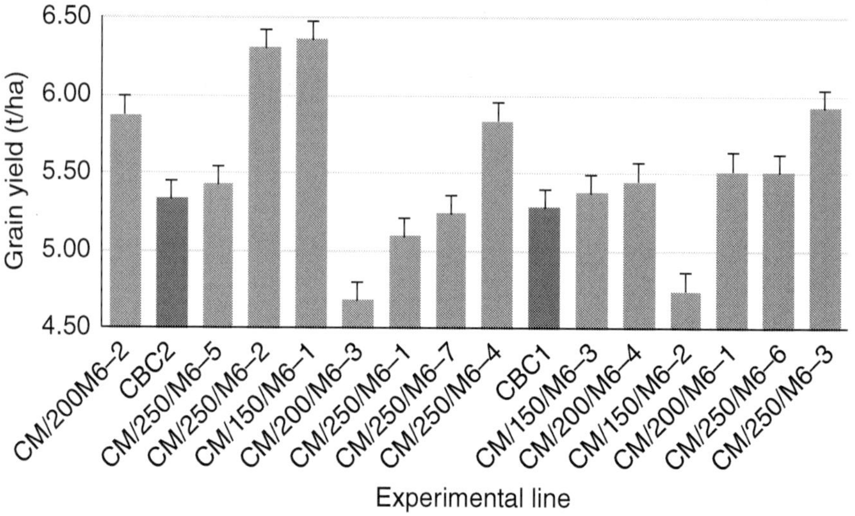

Figure 3. The grain yield of cowpea M_6 experimental lines at three locations in Zimbabwe.

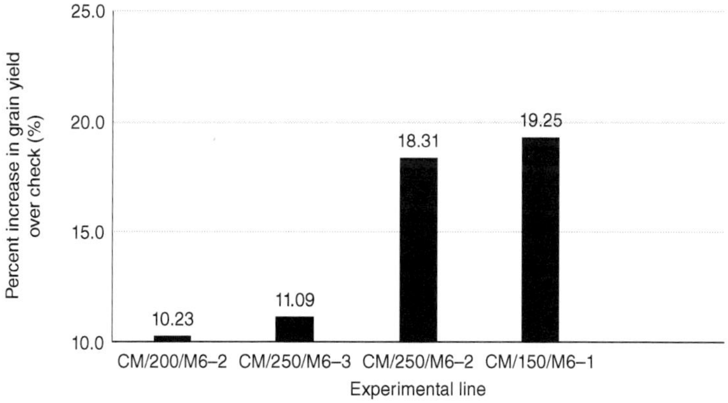

Figure 4. The yield advantage of the best four cowpea M_6 experimental lines over the check cultivar (CBC-2) that were evaluated at the Save Valley Research Station (Zimbabwe) during winter under irrigation.

3.3. Seedling performance of tepary bean mutants

In the study that evaluated the traits that are associated with seedling vigour in tepary bean, the %G declined with increased EMS dose in all the three genotypes, indicating that the chemical mutagen depressed seed germination in tepary bean; hence, the mutagenesis of tepary bean with EMS is unlikely to improve seed germination in the species. 'GEN-6' attained the highest (84.4%) seed germination at 0.5% EMS (v/v) while 'GEN-4' achieved the lowest (48.9%) seed germination at 2.0% EMS (v/v). The highest LD_{50} was estimated to be 3.37% EMS dose (v/v) for 'GEN-3' while 'GEN-6' achieved the lowest (2.26 % EMS dose v/v) (**Table 5**). This suggested that each genotype has a specific optimum dose that induces useful mutations that can be exploited in tepary bean breeding. In addition, the coefficients of determination for each of the linier functions were high (>75%), indicating that there was a notable association between the reduction in seed germination and the concentration of EMS.

Tepary bean genotype	Linear equation	LD_{50} (%EMS)
GEN-3	$y = -13.56x + 95.76$	3.37
GEN-4	$y = -15.98x + 92.88$	2.68
GEN-6	$y = -19.98x + 95.08$	2.26

Table 5. The LD_{50} of three tepary bean genotypes that were treated with ethyl methanesulphonate to induce mutation.

The shoot height (SHT) varied with EMS dose within the genotypes (**Figure 5**). In comparison with the seedlings of the control (0.0% EMS), the SHT in both 'GEN-3' and 'GEN-4' increased by more than 30.0% at the 0.5% EMS but decreased steadily thereafter. In contrast, the SHT in

'GEN-6' was reduced consistently between 0.5 and 1.5% EMS (v/v). Similar studies in other crops also revealed that seedling height decreased with increase in EMS dose [24,25]. With the exception of the PRL, there were significant ($P < 0.05$) differences due to dose effects among the seedlings in all the attributes that were evaluated (**Table 6**). The mean length of the primary roots among the seedlings was >40.0% of the SRL, but on average the SRL was markedly stimulated at 0.5% EMS (v/v).

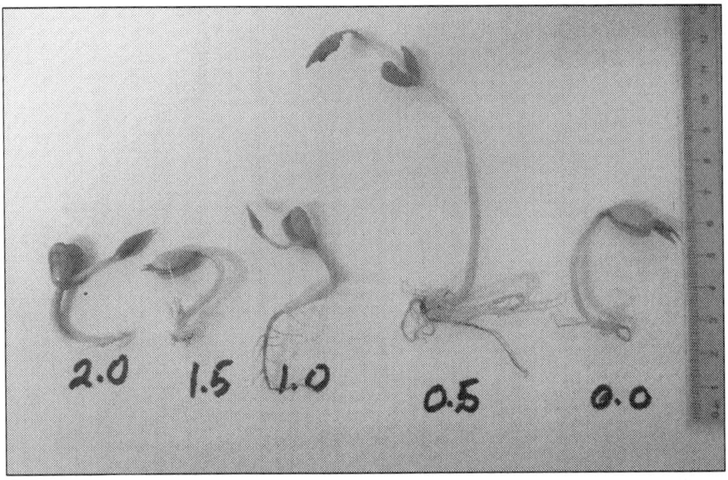

Figure 5. Variation in the shoot height and the number of secondary roots of the tepary bean seedlings within genotypes. (The numbers in bold below each seedling represent the corresponding EMS dose treatment.)

%EMS dose (v/v)	%G	NSR	PRL	SRL	SHT
0.0	100.0 a	20.56 ab	60.22 a	23.22 bc	67.11 a
0.5	79.99 b	30.10 a	53.15 a	68.92 a	83.16 a
1.0	73.32 bc	29.97 a	77.30 a	26.11 b	58.00 ab
1.5	74.16 b	15.92 bc	52.74 a	19.18 bc	34.83 bc
2.0	60.00 c	8.34 c	20.37 b	6.89 c	26.08 c

Means followed by the same letter in each column are not significantly different ($P < 0.05$). [%G = percent seed germination; NSR = number of secondary roots; PRL = primary root length; SRL = secondary root length; SHT = shoot height].

Table 6. The main effects of ethylmethane sulphonate dose on five attributes of seedling vigour in tepary bean.

The number of secondary roots (NSR) generally increased by >45.0% at 0.5 and 1.0% EMS (v/v) dose. Both the maximum (39.0) and lowest (4.0) number of lateral roots were observed for

'GEN-4' at 0.5 and 2.0% EMS (v/v), respectively. In addition, the untreated seedlings of 'GEN-4' developed 50.0% fewer secondary roots than the untreated seedlings of the other two genotypes but trebled the NSR on treatment with 0.5% EMS (v/v) (**Figure 6**). A highly significant ($P < 0.01$) positive linear relationship was observed between the PRL and the NSR. The NSR also showed a positive significant linear relationship with the SHT, indicating that the seedlings which produced many lateral roots also developed relatively tall shoots.

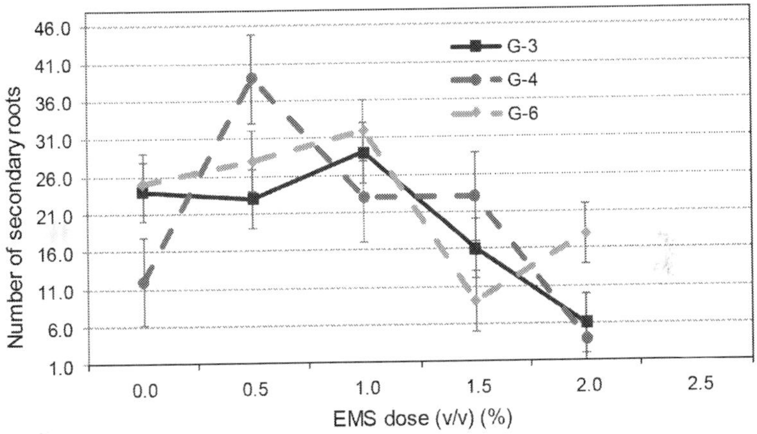

Figure 6. The effect of varying doses of ethyl methanesulphonate on the number of secondary roots in the seedlings of three tepary bean genotypes (G-3 = GEN-3; G-4 = GEN-4; G-6 = GEN-6).

3.4. Field performance of tepary bean mutants

At the adult plant stage, there was a significant ($P < 0.05$) influence of the mutant generation on the NPP, SDW as well as 100-SW. A significant effect of the mutant generation on the NPP was also reported previously in EMS derived horsegram genotypes [28]. The genotype significantly ($P < 0.05$) influenced the PL but not the seed size. Similarly, the dose of EMS showed significant ($P < 0.05$) on both the PL and the seed size. However, the seed size was relatively small (<10.0 g per 100 seeds) compared to the size reported for tepary bean in other studies [29].

Because of the limited number of tepary bean genotypes used in the study, it was difficult to make firm conclusions about its response to EMS, but the results suggested that the mutagen suppresses seed germination and can increase the number of secondary roots in this legume. Therefore, from a plant breeding point of view, the treatment of tepary bean seed with EMS is unlikely to improve seed germination but could increase the number of lateral roots. In previous studies, the number of lateral roots (or profuse branching) and the root length (or capacity for deep rooting) were associated with tolerance to drought in tepary bean or common bean [30–32].

4. Conclusions

These findings provide reference doses for large-scale gamma irradiation of cowpea as well as chemical mutagenesis for tepary bean. In addition, the germplasm produced from these approaches has the potential for selection in a range of agro-ecological conditions across the region, thus creating alternative cropping systems for the smallholder growers. The field trials under irrigation indicated that cowpea can be produced during the off-season, thus providing more options for legume farmers and enhancing food security in the region. In future, it will be interesting to investigate the impact of radiation on the nutritional attributes of these two legumes. In addition, a study of the genetic control of the sensitivity of cowpea to gamma radiation could provide valuable information about its genetic manipulation. The contrast in radio-sensitivity between the cowpea genotypes observed in this study could provide ideal parental combinations for generating segregating progenies for the genetic study of the trait. The effects of mutagenesis using either of the techniques on pest resistance (for instance, to weevils) in diverse germplasm of the two legumes could also be interesting.

Acknowledgements

We wish to thank the IAEA research team at the Joint FAO/IAEA Agriculture and Biotechnology Laboratory, Seibersdorf, Austria. We also express our gratitude to the governments of Namibia and Zimbabwe and the National Research Foundation (South Africa) for funding some of the work reported in this chapter. The authors are grateful to Prof. I.K. Mariga as well as all the farmers who provided some of the germplasm used in this study. We extend a special word of thanks to Mr. Ruzivo Gwata, who generously assisted with various technical aspects of the manuscript. Any reference to a brand name product or organization contained in this chapter does not imply its approval of the product or approval of the authors' views by the organization mentioned herein.

Author details

E. T. Gwata[1], H. Shimelis[2] and P. M. Matova[3]

1 University of Venda, Department of Plant Production, Thohoyandou, Limpopo, South Africa

2 University of KwaZulu-Natal, African Centre for Crop Improvement, Scottsville, South Africa

3 Crop Breeding Institute, Causeway, Harare, Zimbabwe

References

[1] Porch TG, Beaver JS, Brick MA: Registration of tepary germplasm with multiple-stress tolerance, TARS-Tep 22 and TARS-Tep 32. J Plant Reg. 2013;7:358–364.

[2] Rao I, Beebe S, Polania J, Ricaurte J, Cajiao C, Garcia R, Rivera M: Can tepary bean be a model for improvement of drought resistance in common bean? Afr Crop Sci J. 2013;21:265–281.

[3] Shimelis H, Shiringani R: Variance components and heritabilities of yield and agronomic traits among cowpea genotypes. Euphytica. 2010;176:383–389.

[4] Ng O, Marachel R. Cowpea taxonomy, origin, and germplasm. In: Singh SR, Rachie KO, editors. Cowpea research, production and utilization. Chichester: Wiley, 1985. Pp-. 13–21.

[5] Nabhan GP, Felger RS: Teparies in south-western North America. Econ Bot. 1978;32:2–19.

[6] Shisanya CA: Improvement of drought adapted tepary bean (*Phaseolus acutifolius* A. Gray var. *latifolius*) yield through biological nitrogen fixation in semi-arid SE-Kenya. Eur J Agron. 2002;16:13–24.

[7] Ayisi KK, Nkgapele RJ, Dakora FD: Nodule formation and function in six varieties of cowpea (*Vigna unguiculata* L. Walp.) grown in a nitrogen rich soil in South Africa. Symbiosis. 2000;28:17–31.

[8] Ahloowalia BS, Maluszynski M, Nichterlein K: Global impact of mutation-derived varieties. Euphytica. 2002;2:187–204.

[9] Girija M, Dhanavel D: Mutagenic effectiveness and efficiency of gamma rays, ethyl methylmethane sulphonate and their combined treatment in cowpea (*Vigna unguiculata* L. Walp.). Global J Mol Sci. 2009;4:68–75.

[10] Gahlot DR, Vatsa VK, Kumar D: Some mutants for pod and maturity characteristics in M_2 generation of urdbean (*Vigna mungo* (L.) Hepper). Legume Res. 2008;31:272–275.

[11] Manjaya JG, Nandanwar RS: Genetic improvement of soybean variety JS 80–21 through induced mutations. Plant Mut Rep. 2007;1:36–40.

[12] Manigopa-Chakraborty GJ, Singh DN, Virk DS, Prasad SC: Selection in M_2 generation of horsegram (*Macrotyloma uniflorum*) through participatory plant breeding. J Arid-Legumes. 2005;2:1–4.

[13] Wani AA, Anis M: Gamma rays induced bold seeded high yielding mutant in chickpea. Mut Breed Newslett. 2001;45:20–21.

[14] Harding SS, Johnson SD, Taylor DR, Dixon CA, Turay MY: Effect of gamma rays on seed germination, seedling height, survival percentage and tiller production in some rice varieties cultivated in Sierra Leone. Am J Exp Agr. 2012;2:247–255.

[15] Jamil M, Khan UQ: Study of genetic variation in yield components of wheat cultivar Bukhtwar-92 as induced by gamma radiation. Asian J Plant Sci. 2002;5:579–580.

[16] CvejićS, JocićS, ProdanovićS, TerzićS, MiladinovićD, BalalićI: Creating new genetic variability in sunflower using induced mutations. Helia. 2011;34:47–54.

[17] Owoseni O, Okwaro H, Afza R, Bado S, Dixon A, Mba C: Radio-sensitivity and in vitro mutagenesis in African accessions of cassava, *Manihot esculenta* Crantz. Plant Mutat Rep. 2007;1:32–36.

[18] Velasco L, Perez-Vich B, Fernandez-Martinez JM: The role of mutagenesis in the modification of the fatty acid profile of oilseed crops. J Appl Genet. 1999;40:185–209.

[19] Novak FJ, Brunner H: Plant breeding: induced mutation technology for crop improvement. IAEA Bull. 1992;4:24–33.

[20] Horn L, Shimelis H: Radio-sensitivity of selected cowpea (*Vigna unguiculata*) genotypes to varying gamma irradiation doses. Sci Res Ess. 2013;8:1991–1997.

[21] Ndou VN, Shimelis H, Odindo A, Modi AT: Response of selected wheat genotypes to ethylmethane sulfonate concentration, treatment temperature and duration. Sci Res Ess. 2013;8:198–196.

[22] Cobbinah FA, Addo-Quaye AA, Asante IK: Characterization, evaluation and selection of cowpea accessions with desirable traits from eight regions of Ghana. J Agri Biol Sci. 2011;6:21–32.

[23] Animasaun DA, Oyedeji S, Azeez YK, Mustapha OT, Azeez MA: Genetic variability study among ten cultivars of cowpea (*Vigna unguiculata* L. Walp) using morpho-agronomic traits and nutritional composition. J Agri Sci. 2015;10:119–130.

[24] Elangovan R, Pavadai P: Studies on induced chemical mutagenesis in bhendi (*Abelmoschus esculentus* (L.) Moench). Int J Mod Biol Med. 2015;6:30–37.

[25] Sarada C, Uma Jyothi K, Srinivasa Rao V, Reddy PV: Mutagenic sensitivity of gamma rays, EMS and their combinations on germination and seedling vigour in coriander (*Coriandrum sativum* L). Int J Adv Pharm Biol Chem. 2015;4:430–433.

[26] Sikder S, Biswas P, Hazra P, Akhtar S, Chattopadhyay A, Badigannavar AM, D'Souza SF: Induction of mutation in tomato (*Solanum lycopersicum* L.) by gamma irradiation and EMS. Ind J Genet. 2013;73:392–399.

[27] Constantin MJ, Klobe WD, Skold LN: Effects of physical and chemical mutagens on survival, growth, and seed yield of soybeans. Crop Sci. 1976;16:49–52.

[28] Bolbhat SN, Dhumal KN: Effect of mutagens on quantitative characters in M_2 and M_3 generation of horsegram (*Macrotyloma uniflorum*). Int J Sci Res Publ. 2012;2:1–7.

[29] Bhardwaj HL, Rangappa M, Hamama AA: Planting time and genotype effects on tepary bean productivity. Hort Sci. 2002;37:317–318.

[30] Beebe SE, Rao IM, Blair MW, Acosta-Gallegos JA: Phenotyping common beans for adaptation to drought. Front Plant Physiol. 2013;4:1–20.

[31] Butare L, Rao IM, Lepoivre P, Polania J, Cajiao C, Cuasquer J, Beebe S: New genetic sources of resistance in the genus *Phaseolus* to individual and combined aluminium toxicity and progressive soil drying stresses. Euphytica. 2011;181:385–404.

[32] Mohamed MF, Schmitz-Eiberger N, Keutgen N, Noga G: Comparative drought postponing and tolerance potentials of two tepary bean lines in relation to seed yield. Afr Crop Sci J. 2005;13:49–60.

Chapter 5

Tomato Production with Cover Crops in Greenhouse

Hajime Araki

Additional information is available at the end of the chapter

http://dx.doi.org/10.5772/62641

Abstract

One of the ways to reduce chemical fertilizer application is the use of cover crops, which improve soil properties and supply nutrition to subsequent crops. Hairy vetch (*Vicia villosa* R.; HV) is one of the processing legume cover crops. A similar yield of fresh marketable tomato (*Solanum lycopersicum* L.) was obtained in the soil with HV mulch and incorporation even if the reduction of chemical N fertilizer input compared with the conventional production with 240 kg-N/ha fertilizer in the greenhouse from 2006 to 2012. Using 15N-labeling method, HV residue incorporated into soil was decomposed rapidly for about 1 month and N released from HV residue was absorbed into the tomato plant. Nitrogen was absorbed by tomato through out production period. The rate of N uptake derived from HV to total N uptake in tomato plants (%N_{dfhv}) in the small amount N fertilizer was higher than that with high amount of N fertilizer application. It ranged from 24.8% in 240 kg-N/ha to 37.1% in no N fertilizer. The nitrogen use efficiency (NUE) from HV-derived N by tomato plant reached about 50% during the tomato production with HV incorporation. Other 50% of HV-derived N remained in the soil and 4% of were absorbed by tomato in the next year's production. HV has the possibility of alternative material for basal N fertilizer to ensure the tomato growth of early period after transplanting, and continuous supply of N is necessary to late stage of tomato. The combined system of incorporation of HV cultivated at the seeding density of 20–50 kg/ha before tomato planting and the slow released N fertilizer was established for the reduction N fertilizer application and obtaining conventional tomato yield in plastic house.

Keywords: cover cropping, hairy vetch, nitrogen, nitrogen dynamics, tomato

1 Introduction

1.1 Management of fertilizer application in tomato production in plastic house

More than 70% of fruit vegetables including tomato were repeatedly produced with the application of much amount of chemical fertilizer in plastic house in Japan, and salt accumulation and injury by continuous cropping became serious problems. Excessive N input causes extra N accumulation in the soil [1], as a result of environmental pollution, such as nitrate leaching and greenhouse gas emission occur [2]. For the establishment of sustainable greenhouse production, reducing fertilizer inputs and proper applications are required.

Because tomatoes are produced with N application by basal and side-dressing fertilizer in practice, the dynamics of N derived from basal, side-dressing fertilizer, and soil in the plant are complicated, and real-time nutritional diagnosis was developed [3, 4].

Side dressings of fertilizer combined with diagnosis of nutrient conditions are popularly carried out in production areas [4, 5]. Leaf petioles below the first fruit cluster or upper fruit cluster with 2–4 cm size tomatoes are used as material for the nitrate analysis. Nitrate concentration of ca 3000–4000 ppm was reported to be an appropriate concentration for vegetative growth in tomato.

Controlled release fertilizer, the so-called slow-release fertilizer, is applied at the beginning of tomato production to reduce application work. These fertilizer management methods contribute to proper nutrient application in tomato production. However, for sustainable tomato production in greenhouses or plastic houses, soil properties have to be improved and be healthy in addition to proper N fertilization.

1.2 Advantage of cover cropping

Planting a cover crop is one of the biological tools used for sustainable crop production, which has the effects of N supply [6], increasing organic soil carbon [7], improving soil physical properties [8], and so on. Among the various kinds of cover crops, hairy vetch (*Vicia villosa* R.; HV), legume crop, is one of the important species. HV residues can supply plenty of N due to its efficiency in biological nitrogen fixation [9, 10]. HV also has other advantages, such as adaptability to low temperatures, resistance to pests, delaying senescence, covering ground surface effectively, and fitness for vegetable production, particularly in rotation with tomatoes [11]. Araki et al. [7] also reported that utilizing HV could reduce chemical N fertilizer inputs to half of the recommended amount without yield reduction in tomato production. Such results showed that HV had potential as an alternative fertilizer to chemical N fertilizers.

The N release pattern from inorganic or organic fertilizer has to be synchronized with crop demands for proper application [12]. Yaffa et al. [13] have shown the synchronization of tomato N uptake and N release from cover crops; the tomato N uptake increased after the increase of soil inorganic N, followed by a decline. On the other hand, Kumar et al. [11] reported that because N release from white clover residues was faster under rotary hoeing treatment, it was not synchronized with the N demand of wheat during its early growth period and resulted in minimum N-benefits. We have to investigate the N supply pattern when HV was introduced in tomato cropping in plastic house.

Non-legume cover crops are higher in carbon than legume cover crops. Because of their high carbon content, grasses break down more slowly than legumes, resulting in longer-lasting residue. As grasses mature, the carbon-to-nitrogen ratio (C:N) increases. This has two tangible results: The higher carbon residue is harder for soil microbes to break down, so the process takes longer, and the nutrients contained in the cover crop residue usually are less available to the next crop.

2 Tomato production with cover crops, 2006–2012

2.1 Field preparation and chemical fertilizer application

Tomatoes were grown in the rows with or without cover crop residue mulch shown in **Table 1**, in high plastic tunnels, adding nitrogen fertilizer 120 kg and 240 kg/ha, 2006 and 2007.

Date	Operation
March 22	Cover plastic film
April 4	Surface tillage in each row
April 5	Sowing of cover crop
May 26	Mowing of cover crop
	Application of fertilizers
	Making an organic mulch
May 29	Planting of tomato seedings
	Measurement of nitrate in leaf petiole and growth index
July 7–	Tomato harvest every 2–3 days
October 15	
November 16	Measurement of Soil N and C

Source: Araki et al., Hort. Environ.Biotechnol. 50:324-328. 2009.

Table 1. Field operation in the tomato production with cover crop, 2007.

Hairy vetch (*Vicia villosa* R.) and wild oat (*Avena sterigosa* L.) were used for cover crop. They were drill planted at 10–15 cm distance, each alone or together on April 5. Seeding density was 50 kg/ha in hairy vetch, 100 kg/ha in wild oat, and 35 and 50 kg/ha in hairy vetch and wild oat, respectively. Cover crops were grown until May 26 and mowed by cutter 2 cm above the ground surface for making residue mulch of cover crops. The plots with cover crops were left untilled to maintain the residue mulch, and bare plot without cover crops were slightly tilled by hand (**Table 2**, **Figure 1**).

Year Examined	Mark	Cover crop		Fertilizer		
		Spices	Treatment	N^z (kg/ha)	P_2O_5 (kg/ha)	K_2O (kg/ha)
2006–2007	N240	Nothing	Bare	240	200	200
	N120	Nothing	Bare	120	200	200

Year Examined	Mark	Cover crop		Fertilizer		
		Spices	Treatment	N^z (kg/ha)	P_2O_5 (kg/ha)	K_2O (kg/ha)
	HV	HV	Mulch	120	200	200
	Oats	Oats	Mulch	120	200	200
	Mix	HV + oats	Mulch	120	200	200
2008	N240	Nothing	Bare	240	200	200
	N80	Nothing	Bare	80	200	200
	HV	HV	Mulch	80	200	200
	Oats	Oats	Mulch	80	200	200
	Mix	HV + oats	Mulch	80	200	200
2009–2012	N240	Nothing	Bare	240	200	200
	HV	HV	Incorporation	80	200	200
	HV	HV	Mulch	80	200	200
	Oats	Oats	Mulch	80	200	200
	Mix	HV + oats	Mulch	80	200	200

[z]In both N rates, 20 and 80% of total N fertilizer were applied by fast-release (ammonium sulfate) and slow-release fertilizer (LPS100, N40%), respectively.
Source: Araki et al., Hort. Environ. Biotechnol. 50:324-328. 2009.

Table 2. Hairy vetch treatment and fertilizer application in tomato plots from 2006 to 2012.

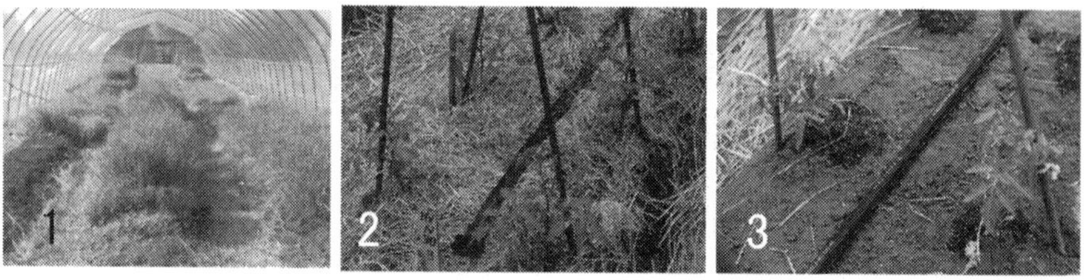

Figure 1. Cover crops grown in plastic high tunnel (1), hairy vetch reside mulch plot (2) and bare plot (3).Source: Araki et al., Hort. Environ. Biotechnol. 50:324–328. 2009.

Chemical fertilizers for tomato were applied on the ground surface on May 27, 2006. Two rates of nitrogen fertilizer of 120 and 240 kg/ha were applied in the bare rows, and 120 kg N/ha fertilizer was done in rows with cover crops. In both N rates, 20 and 80% of total N fertilizer were applied by fast-release (ammonium sulfate) and slow-effect fertilizer (LP40, Chisso ASAHI Co. Ltd.), respectively (**Table 2**). In every plot, 200 kg of P_2O_5 and K_2O was added per ha.

Each plot was 0.8 m wide and 3 m long, 0.6 m between tomato lines and 0.5 m between plants. Planting density was 22,220 plants/ha. Treatments were arranged in a randomized block design with three replications.

Tomato production with cover crops was continued till 2012. N fertilizer application in cover crop plots reduced to 80 kg/ha from 2008, and the plot of HV incorporation was set up from 2009.

2.2 Biomass production of cover crops

Wild oat grew to heading stage; however, seeds were not developed at the mowing time. Flowering occurred in some HV plants. At the mowing, late in May, contents of N and C were 4.3 and 41.3% in HV (C/N: 10.1), and 1.4 and 37.1% in oats (C/N: 32.3) in average from 2007 to 2012 (**Table 3**).

Cover	Concentration		N,C	FW			DW			N Contents (kg/ha)
Crop	N (%)	C (%)	C/N ratio	HV (kg/ha)	Oats (kg/ha)	Total (kg/ha)	HV (kg/ha)	Oats (kg/ha)	Total (kg/ha)	
HV	4.3	41.3	10.1	33,000	-	33,000	4,709		4,709	203
Oats	1.4	37.1	32.3	-	28,270	28,270	-	5,301	5,301	87
Mix				11,570	26,270	37,840	1,595	4,950	6,545	148

Data was the average of values obtained from 2007 to 2012.

Table 3. Biomass production of cover crops, hairy vetch and oats, cultivated in the plastic house for 2 months, April and May. 2007–2012.

Aboveground biomass (dry weight) was 4709 kg/ha in HV and 5301 kg/ha in wild oat late in May. However, in mix-culture, it was 1595 kg/10a in HV and 4950 kg/ha in wild oat.

Sainju et al. [14] reported that bi-culture of legume and non-legume cover crops had greater biomass yield, and also N and C contents in cover crops than monoculture of each species in the southeast area of USA. On the other hand, aboveground and underground biomass yield, and N and C contents of cover crops were varied by year and experimental location.

Experimental location of this examination, Sapporo, Japan, was snow cover region. More than 1 m high snow cover is observed in winter. HV is a typical winter annual legume crops originally, but few plants survive after long snow cover [15]. Wild oat also cannot overwinter under snow cover more than 3 month in Sapporo. HV and wild oat were usually sown in early spring in Sapporo. Greater biomass in bi-culture of wild oat and HV was not observed than monoculture of wild oat because of short growing period of cover crops.

2.3 Tomato growth and yield, 2007

2.3.1 Nitrate in petiole sap

There was a difference in nitrate concentration in petiole sap in leaf below first fruit cluster among treatments in July and August. Nitrate in HV plot showed 3650 and 3550 ppm in July and August (**Figure 2**). Those in Bare + N240 kg plot were 3280 and 2966 ppm, respectively. However, nitrate concentrations in other treatments were smaller than those in HV and Bare + N240 kg plots. That in oat plots was smallest. Though nitrate value decreased from July to August in bare plot (N120 kg), it increased in oat and mix (HV + Oat) plots. Such observation accorded with the result that N content became high in the leaves of tomatoes produced with HV mulch [16].

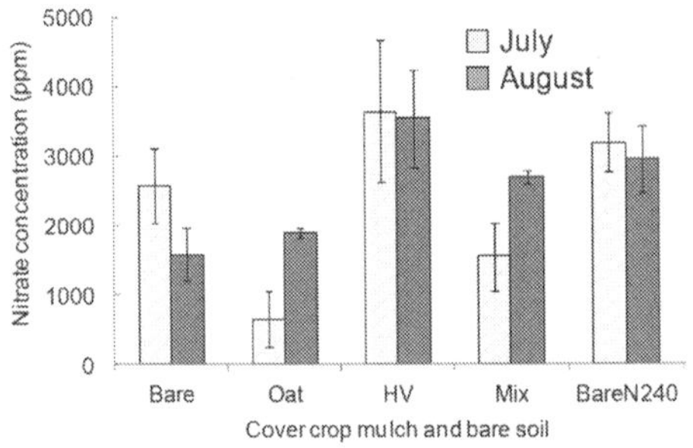

Figure 2. Effect of cover crop residue mulch on nitrate concentration of petiole sap on July 9 and August 10, 2007. 240 kg N fertilizer per ha was added into BareN240 plot and 120 kg N fertilizer per ha was done into other plots. Vertical bars represents SE (n = 3).Source: Araki et al., Hort. Environ. Biotechnol. 50:324–328. 2009.

2.3.2 Growth and yield of tomato

Similar total marketable yield was shown in HV and Bare + N240 kg plots, 78.2 t/ha in the former and 79.5 t/ha in the latter (**Figure 3**). Yield in first and second fruit cluster in Bare + N240 kg plot was larger than those in HV plot. Yields in Bare + N120 kg and mix plots were 68.8 t and 69.6 t/ha, smaller than those in HV and Bare + N240 kg plots. Oat plot showed smallest yield, 61.5 t/ha.

To consider fruit yield, nitrogen absorption/application rate, and nitrate nitrogen concentration, the proper range of petiole sap nitrate concentration was 4000–7000 ppm [4]. This has been recognized as recommendable value of nitrate concentration for current yield in Hokkaido prefecture. In this examination, nitrate concentrations in petiole sap in HV and Bare + N240 kg plots were close to the recommendable value in July and August. These plots have possibility to obtain the current yield. Those in other plots were obviously lower than recommended value, and it is necessary to apply the N fertilizer for the current yield.

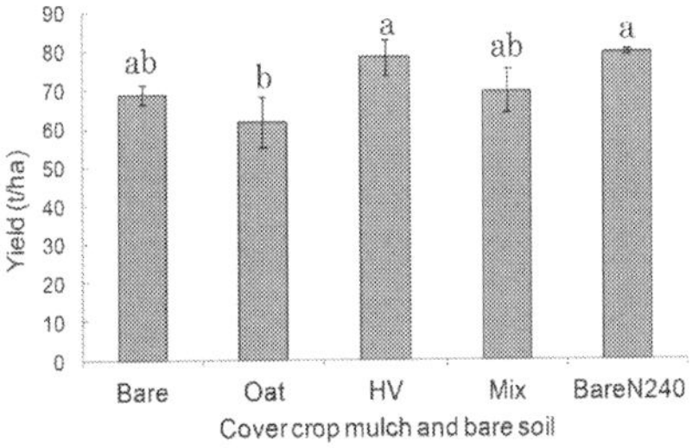

Figure 3. Effect of cover crop residue mulch on total fresh marketable yield of tomato 2007. 24 kg N fertilizer per 10a was added into BareN24 plot and 12 kg N fertilizer per 10a was done into other plots. Vertical bars represent SE (n = 3). Means followed by different letters are significantly different at 5%, Tukey's test.Source: Araki et al., Hort. Environ. Biotechnol. 50:324–328. 2009.

In bare plots, especially adding with N120 kg, nitrate concentration in petiole tended to decrease from July to August; however, it increased in oat and mix plots in spite of same rate of N fertilizer. It is caused by decomposing the organic matter of cover crop residue applied in 2006 and 2007.

Nitrate concentration in petiole sap was concerned with growth index (GI), indicator of vegetative growth. GI values in Bare + N240 kg and HV plots were higher than other cover crop plots. HV, typical legume crops, decomposes faster than non-legume crops because of low C/N ratio [17], and released nitrogen is absorbed into tomato plant. However, C/N ratio of wild oat is high, as much as 24 in our previous observation. Nitrogen absorbance into tomato plants was restricted due to immobilization in soil.

Same trend in marketable tomato yield was observed as GI, with larger yield in Bare + N240 kg and HV plots, medium yield in Bare + N120 kg and mix plots and smallest in oat plots. The examined location is a cool summer region of which air temperature usually decreases from September. It is necessary to obtain good vegetative growth until August for getting much yield.

Even if N fertilizer decreases to half of conventional (240 kg/ha), current tomato yield was obtained in the HV plots. Such tomatoes are recognized as organically grown agro-product in combined with the reduction of fungicide and pesticide application.

2.4 Long-term evaluation of tomato yield, 2007–2012

Such tomato production system continued till 2012 (**Table 4**). The vegetative growth (GI) and marketable yield showed same trend as 2007. That is, highest GI and yield were shown in Bare-N240 plot. However, there was no significant difference between Bare-N240 and HV (N80 kg)-incorporation. GI and marketable yield of HV mulch plot were a little smaller than those of Bare-N240 and HV (N80 kg)-incorporation. From the long-term examination, 2008–2010, it was clarified HV supports the vegetative growth and tomato yield even if N fertilizer reduces to half or one third of conventional application in greenhouse.

Mark (cover crops)	Treatment of cover crops	N fertilizer[y] (kg/ha)	Growth index[x]		Marketable yield (t/10a)	
N240	Bare	240	40514	a[w]	4.7	a
HV	Incorporation	80	38424	a	4.3	a
HV	Mulch	80	33200	b	4.1	a
Oats	Mulch	80	25365	c	2.6	b
Mix	Mulch	80	29.336	bc	3.0	b
Tukey's test[w]			*		*	

[z]Data was average of the values obtained from 2007 to 2012.
[y]In both N rates, 20 and 80% of total N fertilizer were applied by fast-release (ammonium sulfate) and slow-release fertilizer (LPS100), respectively.
[x]Growth index (GI) was measured 6 weeks after transplanting, just before the first harvest.
[w]Means followed by different letters and asterisk are significantly different among the treatments at 5%, Tukey's test. NS: not significant.

Table 4. Effects of cover crops and N fertilizer on the growth and the yield of tomato: 2007–2012[z].

2.5 Soil N and C content after tomato production

Increase of inorganic N increased near soil surface, 0–5 cm depth, in the rows with cover crops in the case of N 120 kg/ha application, 2007. Considering the high nitrate in petiole, high GI and large yield in plots with HV, it is thought that released N from cover crops was absorbed into tomato plants in near soil surface. There was no significant difference in soil total N among the plots though the examination period (**Table 5**).

Mark (cover crops)	Treatment of cover crops	0.5 cm				15 cm			
		N (%)		C (%)		N (%)		C (%)	
		2007	2012	2007	2012	2007	2012	2007	2012
N240	Bare	0.28	0.22	3.89	3.57	0.24	0.22	3.54	3.50
HV	Incorporation	0.24	0.26	3.45	3.51	0.23	0.22	3.35	3.50
HV	Mulch	0.30	0.24	4.24	3.87	0.24	0.23	3.70	3.32
Oats	Mulch	0.27	0.23	4.08	3.69	0.25	0.23	3.57	3.55
Mix	Mulch	0.30	0.27	4.61	4.07	0.26	0.25	3.77	3.78

Data in 2007 and 2012 were presented.

Table 5. Content of total nitrogen and total carbon in the soil of the plot cultivated cover crops for 7 years (2006–2012), at the depth 5 cm and 15 cm.

As to soil carbon, the change of soil C content was observed in of 0–5 cm depth soil because of leaving cover crop residue on the soil surface. There was tendency to increase in mix plot (oats and HV); however, significant difference was recognized only 2 years, 2007 and 2008.

Winter cover crops have the potential to increase soil organic C in agricultural soils [18]. Komatsuzaki and Mu [19] evaluated the effects of tillage in continuous field rice cropping with rye and hairy vetch cover crops in Kanto region, non-snow cover region in Japan. Soil organic carbon in the top soil, 0–2.5 cm depth, increased compared with winter fallow 2 years later adopting cover cropping; however, other soil layer did not show any change in their observation.

Organic matter level in the soils under mixed cover crops improved as much as 8.8% after 3 years of cover crop use [20]. Interestingly, soil under the legume-only cover actually dropped slightly in organic matter content after 3 years, probably because the lower C/N ratio of the incorporated organic matter caused more rapid microbial breakdown. Soil C varies from year-to-year as a result of weather-affected changes in crop residue inputs or decomposition of residues and organic matter [21].

As to one of the reasons of little change of soil C in our examination, ash soil is distributed around plot area and soil C content is originally high, more than 3%. If the examination was performed in the soil with low content of soil C, soil C will increase using of cover crop, especially no legume cover crops. Content of soil C affects the biological properties of soil. Some methods such as active carbon and SIR (substrate-induced respiratory) are applied for the estimation of diversity of microorganisms.

3 N dynamics in tomato production with HV

3.1 Stable isotope technique

These results mentioned previous section showed that HV could be alternative fertilizer for crop production instead of chemical N fertilizer and become a useful tool to solve the high input problem in N management. It is important to clarify the tomato uptake of N mineralized from HV residue for the establishment of effective N management in the cropping system with cover crops.

The method using ^{15}N-labelled plant materials has been effective for direct estimation of N uptake from the cover crops. Earlier studies have found that the N uptake by the subsequent crop was 6–25% of N applied by ^{15}N-labelled cover crops, HV, ryegrass, etc [10, 22–25]. The efficiency differed depending on subsequent crop species, cover crop species, or cultivation circumstances.

In tomato production with cover crops, Thönnissen et al. [26] reported that when legumes were incorporated or mulched into the soil, tomato absorbed 8.9 or 9.6% of soybean-derived N and 10.0 or 15.0% of indigofera-derived N, respectively. In other report, the higher recovery rate of cover crop-derived N was also reported; 56% of HV-derived N was recovered by rice [27]. ^{15}N-labeling method was used in the evaluation of N recovery from cover crops in these reports.

The application effect of legume cover crop, hairy vetch (*Vicia villosa* R.; HV), on N dynamics in fresh market tomato (*Solanum lycopersicum* L.), "House Momotaro," was investigated using

^{15}N-labelling method [28]. Tomato seedlings were transplanted in the 1/2000a Wagner pot at 0, 80, 240 kg ha^{-1} of N application (N0HV, N80HV and N240HV) on June 9. Before transplanting, the labeled HV (0.86 atom% excess) and chemical fertilizer were incorporated into soil.

3.2 Absorption and distribution N derived from HV

HV-derived N uptake was recognized mainly in first 4 WAT. Especially, in N240HV, the uptake of HV-derived N ceased at 4 WAT. The uptake amounts of HV-derived N at 10 WAT were 587, 657, and 729 mg plant^{-1} in N240HV, N80HV, and N0HV, respectively, and there were significant differences among three treatments (**Figure 4**). The ratio of N uptake derived from HV to total N uptake in tomato plants (%N_{dfhv}) was the highest at 2 WAT, and %N_{dfhv} in N80HV (52.1%) and N0HV (51.5%) were significantly higher than in N240HV (43.6%) (**Figure 5**). After 2 WAT, %N_{dfhv} was decreased gradually in all N rates as tomatoes grew, and it was decreased to 24.8, 34.4, and 37.1% in N240HV, N80HV, and N0HV, respectively, until 12 WAT (**Figure 6**). The nitrogen use efficiency (NUE) by tomato plant from HV-derived N was the highest at 10 WAT, and N0HV (55.3%) was significantly higher than N240HV (44.5%) and N80HV (49.8%) (**Table 5**).

The partition rate of HV-derived N into fruits was 63.9 and 39.7% of HV-derived N was partitioned into low fruit clusters, first and second. The partition rate of N derived from soil and fertilizer into fruits was 57.9%, significantly lower than that of HV-derived N. From these results, it was clarified that (1) HV-derived N was used effectively in small rate of chemical N fertilizer and (2) the N supply effect from HV was expressed in early period of tomato growth (**Table 6**).

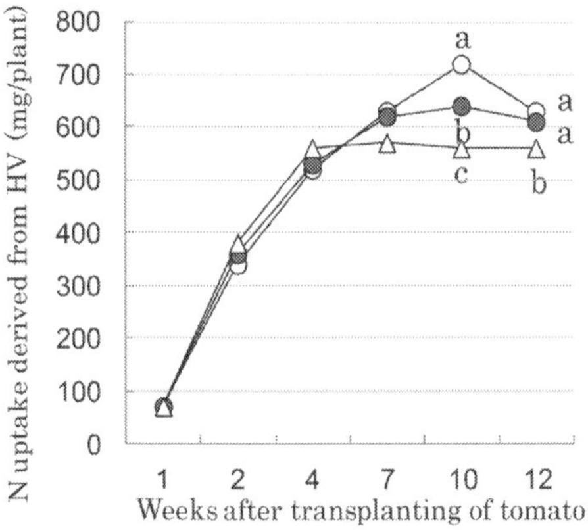

Figure 4. Effect of N fertilizer and HV treatment on the increase of the amount of tomato plant N uptake derived from HV. The plots of N0HV (○), N80HV (●), and N240HV (Δ) were fertilized 0, 80, and 240 kg N ha^{-1}, respectively, and applied HV (1319 mgN pot^{-1}). Means followed by different letters are significantly different at 5%, Tukey's test.Source: Sugihara et al., J. Japan. Soc. Hort. Sci. 82: 30–38. 2013. Available online at www.jstage.jst.go.jp/browse/jjshs1

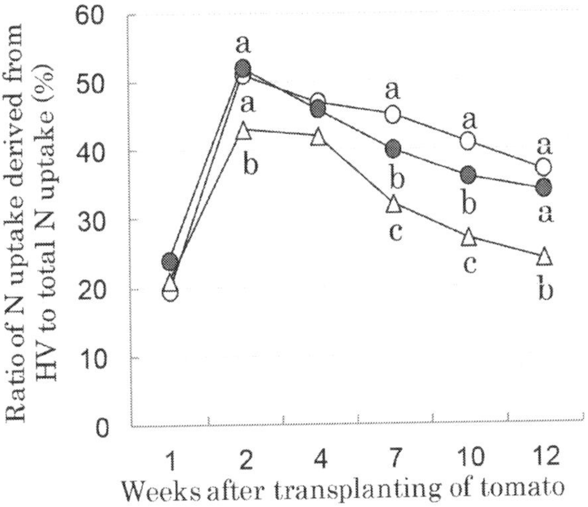

Figure 5. Effect of N fertilizer and HV treatment on the change of the ratio of plant N uptake derived from HV to total N uptake. The plots of N0HV (○), N80HV (●), and N240HV (Δ) were fertilized 0, 80 and 240 kg N ha^{-1}, respectively, and applied HV (1319 mgN pot^{-1}). Means followed by different letters are significantly different at 5%, Tukey's test.Source: Sugihara et al., J. Japan. Soc. Hort. Sci. 82: 30–38. 2013. Available online at www.jstage.jst.go.jp/browse/jjshs1

Treatment[z]	Nitrogen use efficiency (%)							
	Weeks after transplant (WAT)							
	1	2	4	7	10		12	
N240HV	5.1	29.4	43.4	45.2	44.5	c[y]	44.4	b
N80HV	4.8	27.8	41.2	48.7	49.8	b	47.5	ab
N0HV	4.4	25.9	40.3	49.9	55.6	a	49.4	a
Tukey's test[y]	ns[y]	ns	ns	ns	*		*	

[z]The plots of N240HV, N80HV and N0HV were fertilized 240, 80 and 0 kg N ha^{-1}, respectively, and applied HV (1,319mgN pot^{-1}).
[y]Means followed by different letters and asterisk are significantly different among the treatments at 5%, Tukey's test. NS: not significant.
Source: Sugihara et al., J. Japan. Soc. Hort. Sci. 82: 30-38. 2013. Available online at www.jstage.jst.go.jp/browse/jjshs1

Table 6. Effect of N fertilizer and HV treatment on nitrogen use efficiency (NUE) derived from HV.

3.3 Combination of N fertilizer, HV, fast-release N and slow-release N

In order to improve the use efficiency of both hairy vetch (*Vicia villosa* R.; HV) and chemical N fertilizer, N release and uptake patterns from HV, fast-release N fertilizer (FF), and slow-release N fertilizer (SF) in fresh market tomato (*Solanum lycopersicum* L.) production were investigated using the ^{15}N-labeling method. There was no difference in tomato fruit yield between FF + SF and SF-only. HV-derived N was up taken by the tomatoes mainly until 4 weeks after transplant (WAT). The uptake amount of HV-derived N (N_{dfhv}) was same in the pot with FF + SF and SF-only. The rate of N uptake derived from HV to total N uptake in tomato plants (%N_{dfhv}) was 43% (480/1116 mg) in SF-only, higher than that in FF + SF(35%, 430/1204 mg) at 4 WAT; however, such difference disappeared after 4 WAT (**Table 7**). N uptake by tomato plants was continued 12 WAT. From these results, HV has possibility of alternative material for FF to ensure the tomato growth of early period after transplanting and continuous supply of N is necessary to late stage of tomato.

Treatments[z]	N uptake (mg/plant)												
	2 WAT[y]			4 WAT			8 WAT			12 WAT			
	Total[x]	N_{dfhv}	N_{dfhv}	Total	N_{dfsf}	N_{dfhv}	Total	N_{dfsf}	N_{dfhv}	Total		N_{dfsf}	N_{dfhv}
N240HV (FF + SF)	767	508	259	1204	774	430	2010	1518	492	2497	a[w]	1983	a 513
N240HV (SF-only)	745	419	326	1116	636	480	1930	1435	495	2497	a	1959	a 538
N240 (FF + SF)	–	–	–	–	–	–	–	–	–	1748	b	1748	b –
N240(SF-only)	–	–	–	–	–	–	–	–	–	1786	b	1786	b –
t-test	NS[v]	*	NS	NS	*	NS	NS	NS	NS	–		–	NS
Tukey's test	–	–	–	–	–	–	–	–	–	*		*	–

[z]Plots of N240HV were fertilized with 240 kg N·ha^{-1}, and HV was applied (1007 mg N/pot^{-1}). Plots of N240 were fertilized with 240 kg N·ha^{-1} without HV. (FF + SF) contained 20% fast-release fertilizer + 80% slow-release fertilizer, and (SF-only) contained 100% slow-release fertilizer.
[y]WAT: weeks after transplant.
[x]Total = N_{dfsf} + N_{dfhv}, N_{dfsf}; N derived from soil and fertilizer, N_{dfhv}; N derived from HV.
[w]Means followed by different letters and asterisk are significantly different among the treatments at 5%, *t*-test and Tukey's test. NS: Not significant.
Source: Sugihara et al., J. Japan. Soc. Hort. Sci. 83: 222–228. 2014. doi: 10.2503/jjshs1.CH-061

Table 7. Effects of N fertilizer and HV treatments on N uptake by tomato plants.

3.4 Absorption of HV-N remained in soil in the following year

After the tomato cultivation in 2011, the soil was stored in a greenhouse without any water and fertilizer. Tomatoes were cultivated again in the Wagner pots in which contained used soil of 2011 and were added same rate of N fertilizer (0, 80, and 240 kg ha^{-1} of N) and unlabeled HV (935 mgN/pot) in 2012. Total N uptake of tomato plant was higher in N240HV (2377 mg/plant), followed by N80HV (1760 mg/plant), N0HV (1498 mg/plant). On the other hand, the uptake of N derived from HV applied in 2011 (HV_{2011}, 1319 mgN/pot) was not different among the treatments (57.7 mg/plant on average), so nitrogen use efficiency derived from HV_{2011} in 2012 was 4.4% on average (**Figure 6**). This value was much lower than that in 2011 (47.1% on average), but HV_{2011}-N also remained in the soil yet after the tomato cultivation in 2012 (500 mgN/pot). These results showed that although the N supplying effect of HV was small in the following year, HV could be available for not only short-term N source, but also long-term N

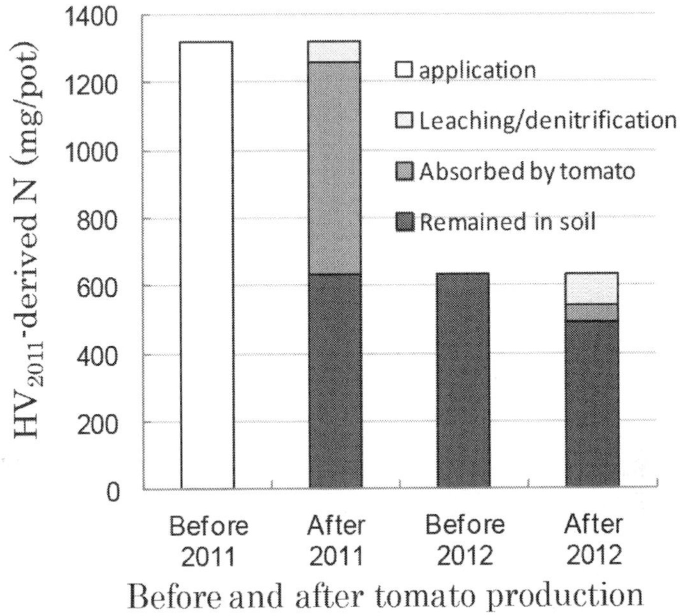

Figure 6. Dynamics of HV_{2011}-N's input and output. The values show an average of three treatments.Source: Sugihara et al., The Horticulture Journal 2016 (preview). doi:10.2503/hortj.MI-073

source, and HV-derived N applied in the previous year was absorbed by tomato plant during relatively early growth period in the following year.

HV-derived N is probably available as alternate of fast-release fertilizer, but in order to cultivate tomato healthy, it is supposed that the application of additional fertilizers for late period growth is needed. Although reducing chemical fertilizer application improves the HV-derived N use efficiency, the excess reducing fertilizer could lead to nitrogen deficiency during late period. Therefore, it is important to balance reducing chemical fertilizers and ensuring normal tomato fruit yield in order to establish the low input sustainable cropping system using HV as a cover crop in tomato cultivation.

From the experiment 2012, the N derived from HV applied in the previous year contributed slightly to the tomato growth, especially in the early growth stage. Although the contribution rate of N derived from HV applied in the previous year was much lower than that from HV applied in the current year, it was suggested that HV could be used for not only short-term N source but also long-term N source as same as other organic materials. The result of this study will be able to use as one of the knowledge to establish the HV-tomato rotation cropping system.

4 Proof study of tomato production with HV

The positive responses of tomatoes grown under hairy vetch residues have economic and environmental importance. From the results mentioned above, HV has the possibility of alternative material for basal N fertilizer to ensure the tomato growth of early period after transplanting and continuous supply of N is necessary to late stage of tomato. A proof study to utilize HV in a real house is necessary because the examinations on N dynamics were carried out in Wagner pot.

4.1 Fertilizer design

The application of ammonium sulfate (AS; 100-N kg/ha), HV (two seeding density; 20 kg and 50 kg/ha) and nothing, was for basal fertilizer management (**Table 8**). AS was applied into soil, May 31, 2015, the previous day of tomato planting. HV grew for over 2 months; it was mowed in late May. At the mowing time, flowering was observed in some plants. Aboveground biomass (dry weight) of HV at densities 50 and 20 kg/ha were 7.2 and 5.9 t/ha, respectively. This biomass accounts for the incorporation of organic nitrogen of 252 and 309 kg/ha of equivalency into soil in HV20 and HV50, respectively. The C:N ratio of HV was low, 9.6, suggesting rapid decomposition and mineralization of organic residues after incorporation into soil.

LPS100 (Long player N fertilizer, slow release type, Chisso ASAHI Co. Ltd) was added in all plots for side dressing. Similarly, in every plot, 200 kg/ha of P_2O_5 as fused magnesium phosphate and 200 kg/ha of K_2O as potassium sulfate were added. Transplanting occurred on June 1, 2015.

Fertilizer or hairy vetch	Basal N		Top N LPS100	Yield of marketable	
	HV seeding (kg/ha)	AS-N application (kg/ha)	application (kg/ha)	tomato (t/ha)	
Control	0	0	150	97	c
AS100	0	100	150	114	b
HV20	20	0	150	129	a
HV50	50	0	150	130	a

Yield means followed by different letters are significantly different among the treatments at 5%, Tukey's test.

Table 8. Design of nitrogen application using HV and chemical fertilizer and marketable yield of fresh tomato.

4.2 Soil inorganic nitrogen and tomato yield

AS100 plots exhibited the highest soil inorganic nitrogen (9 mg/100 g) in the second week after transplanting (2 WAT); however, it showed a decreasing trend (**Table 9**). The soil inorganic nitrogen in HV20 and HV50 plots got to increase from 4 WAT until 6 WAT.

Plots	Inorganic nitrogen (mg/100g)		
	WAT		
	2	6	12
Control	2.6	3.1	1.0
AS100	9.0	3.1	1.1
HV2	2.8	5.0	1.6
HV5	5.4	4.0	2.1

Table 9. Change of inorganic nitrogen in the after tomato planting.

Similar and higher marketable yields were found in HV plots, 130 t/ha in HV50 and 129 t/ha in HV20. These yields were higher than those in AS100 and control plots,114 and 97 t/ha, respectively (**Table 8**).

Because of high N accumulation, HV increased soil inorganic nitrogen, tomato yield, and N uptake [29]. The HV residues increased soil inorganic N in the early stages of tomato cultivation. HV released more nitrogen in the first 6 weeks while ammonium sulfate provided more nitrogen in the first 4 weeks after transplanting. The results were in agreement with previous studies [28, 30–32]. The increased level of inorganic N with the HV at 15– 42 days after residue incorporation may indicate that hairy vetch is suitable to be used as N source for the early stages of tomato cultivation.

From this study, 40% of conventional N fertilizers were reduced by incorporating hairy vetch residues in soil, even though good vegetative growth and high marketable yield were obtained.

Acknowledgements

The author thanks to technical staff of Experiment Farm, Field Science Center for Northern Biosphere, Hokkaido University, for their managing the cover crop and tomato production. The author also thanks to Mr. Y. Sugihara and Mr. R. A. Muchanga, Master course students, Graduated school of Environmental Science, Hokkaido University, for carrying out the examination.

Author details

Hajime Araki*

Address all correspondence to: araki@fsc.hokudai.ac.jp

Field Science Center for Northern Biosphere, Hokkaido University, Kita-ku, Sapporo, 060-0811 , Japan

References

[1] Hao Z. P., Christie P., Zheng F., Li J. L., Chen Q., Wang J. G. and Li X. L. 2009. Excessive nitrogen inputs in intensive greenhouse cultivation may influence soil microbial biomass and community composition. Commun. Soil Sci. Plant Anal. 40:2323–2337.

[2] McNeal B. L., Stanley C. D., Graham W. D., Gilreath P. R., Downey D. and Creighton J. F. 1995. Nutrient loss trends for vegetable and citrus fields in west central Florida, I: Nitrate. J. Environ. Qual. 24:95–100.

[3] Yamada R., Kato T., Ido Y., Seki M. and Hayakawa I. 1995. Rational manuring management of greenhouse tomatoes based on real-time nutritional diagnosis of plant and soil 1. Diagnostic standard according to nitrate concentration of petiole juice. Res. Bull. Aichi Agric. Res. Cent. 27:205–211.

[4] Sakaguchi M., Hikasa Y. and Nakazumi H. 2004. Diagnostic technique for nitrogen nutrition of summer–autumn harvest culture green-house tomato, Japan. J. Soil Sci. Plant Nutr. 75:29–35.

[5] Tanaka T. 2003. Nutritional diagnosis indicator in drip-fertigation on tomato plants in greenhouse culture. Res. Bull. Aichi Agric. Res. Cent. 35:73–78.

[6] Ruffo M. L. and Bollero G. A. 2003. Modeling rye and hairy vetch residue decomposition as a function of degree-days and decomposition-days. Agron. J. 95:900–907.

[7] Araki H., Hane S., Hoshino Y. and Hirata T. 2009. Cover crop use in tomato production in plastic high tunnel. Hortic. Environ. Biotechnol. 50:1–5.

[8] Blevins R. L. and Frye W. W. 1993. Conservation tillage: An ecological approach to soil management. Adv. Agron. 51:33–78

[9] Acosta J. A. A., Amado T. J. C., Neergaard A., Vinther M., Silva L. S. and Nicoloso R. S. 2011. Effect of ^{15}N-labeled hairy vetch and nitrogen fertilization on maize nutrition and yield under no-tillage. R. Bras. Ci. Solo. 35:1337–1345.

[10] Seo J. H., Meisinger J. J. and Lee H. J. 2006. Recovery of nitrogen-15-labeled hairy vetch and fertilizer applied to corn. Agron. J. 98:245–254.

[11] Kumar V., Abdul-Baki A. A., Anderson J. D. and Mattoo A. K. 2005. Cover crop residues enhance growth, improve yield, and delay leaf senescence in greenhouse-grown tomatoes. HortScience. 40:1307–1311.

[12] Kramer A. W., Doaneb T. A., Horwath W. R. and van Kessel C. 2002. Combining fertilizer and organic inputs to synchronize N supply in alternative cropping systems in California. Agric. Ecosyst. Environ. 91:233–243.

[13] Yaffa S., Sainju U. M., Singh B. P. and Reddy K. C. 2000. Fresh market tomato yield and soil nitrogen as affected by tillage, cover cropping, and nitrogen fertilization. HortScience. 35:1258–1262.

[14] Sainju U. M., Whitehead W. F. and Singh B. P. 2005. Biculture legume–cereal cover crops for enhanced biomass yield and carbon and nitrogen. Agron. J. 97:1403–1412.

[15] Araki H., Hatano Y., Horimoto S., Fujii Y and Ito M. 2007. Biomass production and weed control in some winter cover crops in Hokuriku district. Japan. J. Farm. Work. Res. 42:111–122.

[16] Abdul-Baki A. A., Teasdale J. R. and Korcak R. F. 1997. Nitrogen requirements of fresh-market tomatoes on hairy vetch and black polyethylene mulch. HortScience. 32(2):217–221.

[17] Ranells N. N. and Wagger M. G. 1996. Nitrogen release from grass and legume cove r crop monocultures and bicultures. Agron. J. 88:777–782.

[18] Jarecki M. K. and Lal R. 2003. Crop management for soil carbon sequestration. Crit. Rev. Plant. Sci. 22:471–502.

[19] Komatsuzaki M. and Mu Y. 2005. Effects of tillage system and cover cropping on carbon and nitrogen dynamics. Proceeding and abstract of ecological analysis and control of greenhouse gas emission from agriculture in Asia. September 2005, Ibaraki, Japan, pp. 62–67.

[20] Gliessman S. R. 1987. Species interactions and community ecology in low external-input agriculture. Am. J. Altern. Agric. 11:160–165.

[21] Campbell C. A., Zenter R. P., Selles F., Biederbeck V. O., McConkey B. G., Blomert B. and Jefferson P. G. 2000. Quantifying short-term effects of crop rotations on soil organic carbon in south western Saskatchewan. Can. J. Soil. Sci. 80:193–202.

[22] Bergström L. and Kirchmann H. 2004. Leaching and crop uptake of nitrogen from nitrogen-15-labeled green manures and ammonium nitrate. J. Environ. Qual. 33:1786–1792.

[23] Harris G. H., Hesterman O. B., Paul E. A., Peter S. E. and Janke R. R. 1994. Fate of legume and fertilizer nitrogen-15 in a long-term cropping systems experiment. Agron. J. 86:910–915.

[24] Jackson L. E. 2000. Fate and losses of nitrogen from a nitrogen-15-laveled cover crop in an intensively managed vegetable system. Soil. Sci. Soc. Am. J. 64:1404–1412.

[25] Kumar K, Goh. K. M, Scott W. R. and Frampton C. M. 2001. Effects of 15N-labelled crop residues and management practices on subsequent winter wheat yields, nitrogen benefits and recovery under field conditions. J. Agric. Sci. 136:35–53.

[26] Thönnissen C., Midmore D. J., Ladha J. K., Holmer R. J. and Schmidhalter U. 2000. Tomato crop response to short-duration legume green manures in tropical vegetable system. Agron. J. 92:245–253.

[27] Asagi N. and Ueno H. 2009. Nitrogen dynamics in paddy soil applied with various ^{15}N-labelled green manures. Plant. Soil. 322:251–262.

[28] Sugihara Y., Ueno H., Hirata T. and Araki H. 2013. Uptake and distribution of nitrogen derived from hairy vetch used as a cover crop by tomato plant. J. Jpn. Soc. Hortic. Sci. 82:30–38.

[29] Sainju U. M., Singh B. P. and Yaffa S. 1999. Tomato yield and soil quality as influenced by tillage, cover cropping, and nitrogen fertilization. In Hook J. E. (ed.). Proceedings of the 22nd Annual Southern Conservation Tillage Conference for Sustainable Agriculture. Tifton, GA.

[30] Stute J. K. and Posner J. L. 1995. Synchrony between legume nitrogen release and corn demand in the upper Midwest. Agron. J. 87:1063–1069.

[31] Kuo S., Sainju U. M. and Jullum E. J. 1997. Winter cover cropping influence on nitrogen in soil. Soil Sci. Soc. Am. J. 61:1392–1399.

[32] Sainju U. M., Singh B. P. and Whitehead W. F. 2000. Cover crops and nitrogen fertilization effect on soil carbon and nitrogen and tomato yield. Can. J. Soil Sci. 80:523–532.

Chapter 6

Hydroponic Cultivation of Tomato

Bartosz Markiewicz, Tomasz Kleiber and
Maciej Bosiacki

Additional information is available at the end of the chapter

http://dx.doi.org/10.5772/62263

Abstract

Mineral substrates used in plant hydroponic cultures should have low contents of the solid phase and good, stable air and water properties. Rockwool is a substrate with such properties, and it has been produced for plant culture systems since 1969 by I/S H.J. Henriksen and V. Kähler (Denmark). The aim of the study is to evaluate the effect of an application of increasing manganese (Mn) and boron (B) concentrations added to a nutrient solution on the yielding, content of macro- and micronutrients in tomato leaves and fruits (*Lycopersicon esculentum* Mill., cv. Alboney F1 and Emotion F1). Plants were grown in rockwool using a nutrient solution with the following content of Mn (mg dm^{-3}): 0.06, 0.3, 0.6, and 1.2 mg dm^{-3} (Experiment I, 2008–2011) and 2.4, 4.8, 9.6, and 19.2 mg dm^{-3} (Experiment II, 2012)—designated the symbols for Mn: Mn-0, Mn-0.3, Mn-0.6, Mn-1.2, Mn-2.4, Mn-4.8, Mn-9.6, and Mn-19.2 and for B: (0.011), 0.4, 0.8, 1.6 in the form of $Na_2B_4O_7{\cdot}10H_2O$ (Experiment I) and boric acid H_3BO_3 (Experiment II) (combinations of the designated symbols, respectively, B-I, B-II, B-III, and B-IV). The influence of Mn and B nutrition on biometric parameters and chemical composition of leaves and fruits of tomato is discussed.

Keywords: *Lycopersicon esculentum* Mill., rockwool, plant nutrition, manganese, boron

1. Introduction

Due to the quantitatively and qualitatively inferior plant yielding, conventional field cultivation of tomato using fertilizer broadcasting and irrigation is less economically viable in comparison with advanced soilless cultivation systems [1]. Such cultures may be run either applying fertigation (hydroponics) or without it [2] (**Figure 1**).

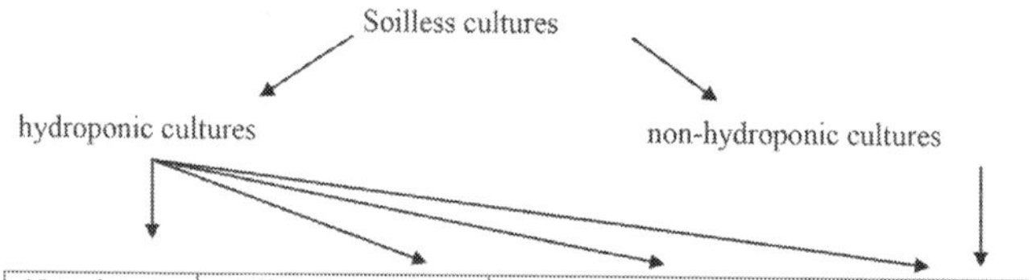

No substrate	Mineral substrate	Synthetic substrates	Organic substrates
Static solution hydroponic system	rockwool (i)	polyurethane foam (i)	peat
NFT	glass wool (i)	polyphenol foam (i)	coir
Aeroponics	expanded clay (i)	Biolaston (i)	bark
	perlite (i)	amine foam (i)	straw
	volcanic lava (i)		lignite
	gravel (i)		sawdust
	sand (i)		wood fiber
	vermiculite		coconut husks
	zeolite		cacao shells

(i)– inert media

Figure 1. Classification of soilless cultures [2].

In horticultural practice, the applications of cultures without a conventional substrate are found, namely aeroponic systems (in which the air is the medium for growth of plant root systems—as the isolated space, periodically filled with injected nutrient solution) [3], the nutrient film technique (NFT; in which a thin film of the surrounding medium is the root growth medium), and the static hydroponic system [4]. In soilless cultures, mineral, synthetic, and organic substrates are used [2,5]. However, currently, mineral substrates, e.g. rockwool, are becoming increasingly popular, among other things, thanks to the precision of plant nutrition in comparison with cultures run in organic substrates, e.g. a mixture of peat and bark or sawdust [6]. Mineral substrates used in plant hydroponic cultures should have low contents of the solid phase and good, stable air and water properties. Rockwool is a substrate with such properties, and it has been produced for plant culture systems since 1969 by I/S H.J. Henriksen and V. Kähler (Denmark). Rockwool, classified to the group of mineral substrates, is produced by melting a natural rock mixture, composed of diabase (60%) and calcium (20%) with coke (20%) at a temperature of 1500–1600°C. Next from such lava rockwool of 0.5 mm in diameter is formed in spinners; it is cooled with air to 200°C; phenolic resins are added (up to 1.3 mg·10 g^{-1} d.m. rockwool) along with binders; and compounds facilitating moisture absorption, providing it with hydrophilic properties. Such prepared rockwool is pressed to form blocks of different sizes, growing mats (e.g. 100 × 20 × 7.5—typically used in cucumber growing; 100 × 15 × 7.5—usually used in tomato culture) or culture cubes for seedling production (e.g. 10 × 10 × 10 cm). Rockwool substrate, thanks to the ultrahigh temperature at which it is produced, is free from pathogens and pests. Companies producing rockwool offer substrates composed of one and two layers, differing in their air and water properties. The fiber arrangement has a significant effect on the distribution of water and electric conductivity (EC) in the growing mat because increasing fiber density in the upper section of the mat has an advantageous effect on nutrient medium permeation and thus facilitates a more uniform growth of plant root systems.

At present, rockwool is commonly used in cultivation of various plant species, both vegetables (such as cucumber and tomato) and ornamental plants (such as rose and gerbera). Its primary advantages include low bulk density (depending on the type ranging from 50 to 100 $g \cdot dm^{-3}$) and high overall porosity (92–98%). Rockwool, in contrast to most organic substrates, ensures uniform air and water conditions and the distribution of the nutrient solution within the root systems of plants, which is important in the case of commercial-scale production. Its important advantage is also connected with preventing the development of anaerobic conditions in the root hair zone, through retention of 20% air at total water capacity. Physical properties of growing mats are as follows: water 52%, the solid phase 3%, and air 45% [7]. However, such properties as water retention or air capacity undergo significant changes upon the completion of the plant vegetation cycle [8].

Rockwool is an inert substrate, devoid of the sorption complex, in which no ion exchange may take place. Its chemical composition may be as follows: P_2O_5 0.2–0.9%, K_2O 0.7–1.3%, CaO 17.5–21.2%, MgO 5.2–9.0%, Fe_2O_3 6.4–8.4%, MnO 0.1–0.5%, Na_2O 1.2–2.2%, SiO_2 40.7–42.9%, Al_2O_3 17.8–19.4%, TiO_2 0.7–2.5%, As < 4 $mg \cdot kg^{-1}$, Cd < 0.5 $mg \cdot kg^{-1}$, Pb < 10 $mg \cdot kg^{-1}$, and Hg < 0.01 $mg \cdot kg^{-1}$. Rockwool also exhibits no buffer properties [9]. It is an alkaline substrate (pH in H_2O = 7.0–8.0), and its reaction is determined by high contents of alkaline elements (Ca, Mg, Na, and K). The high Ca content may cause retrogradation, i.e. chemical sorption of phosphorus. To prevent chemical sorption of nutrients by rockwool before the onset of plant culture, it is acidified with a nutrient solution with pH 5.5–6.0.

An advantage of the application of rockwool as a substrate in plant culture is connected with the limited spread of root system diseases because plants are grown in separate, foil-covered growing mats (as a rule with two plants per mat). A potential risk of diseases may be increased in the case of closed systems with nutrient solution recirculation (in which the nutrient solution leaking from the root systems is recycled for fertigation), at potential problems with its effective disinfection. Applicable nutrient solution disinfection methods in practice include thermal methods [10,11], filtration based on reverse osmosis or another type of membrane systems [12,13], UV radiation, or ozone treatment [14,15].

A disadvantage of rockwool as a homogeneous substrate for plant growing is connected with its problematic disposal and management because this substrate is not biodegradable. It is estimated that from 150 to 200 m^3 rockwool remains after 1-hectare culture of greenhouse tomato [16]. However, such substrates may be used to improve physical properties of soils, particularly heavy soils [8,17], or as an additive to mixed substrates [18]. A certain drawback —in view of the problems with water quality in Europe—may also be connected with the quality requirements for the chemical composition of water for the preparation of fertigation nutrient solutions. Maximum ion concentrations in water may not exceed concentrations recommended for a given plant species (the so-called hydroponic concentrations), taking into consideration the optimal value of EC [19]. In turn, locally observed deterioration of water quality affecting its applicability in fertigation may be connected with both macro- and micronutrients. Response of tomato grown in rockwool to varied concentrations of micronutrients (Mn and B) in nutrient media is presented in the successive chapters.

A serious problem in cultures run in open systems with no nutrient solution recirculation may also be connected with contamination of the natural environment with excess drainage water leaking from the root zone [20]. The greatest contamination is caused by intensive tomato cultures in rockwool run in open systems, which may be as follows: N–NO_3 (up to 245 kg·month·ha^{-1}), K (up to 402 kg·month·ha^{-1}), Ca (up to 145 kg·month·ha^{-1}), and S–SO_4 (up to 102 kg·month·ha^{-1}), while in the case of micronutrients: Fe (up to 2.69 kg·month·ha^{-1}), Mn (up to 0.19 kg·month·ha^{-1}), Zn (up to 0.52 kg·month·ha^{-1}), and Cu (up to 0.09 kg·month·ha^{-1}). In view of the above, apart from studies aiming at the optimization of nutrition for plants grown in rockwool, studies are also being conducted on the applicability of alternative substrates in plant growing to replace rockwool, such as coir, wood fiber, or aeroponic systems [5,21–24].

2. The influence of selected micronutrient nutrition on plant yielding

2.1. Manganese

2.1.1. The physiological role

Mn, similarly iron (Fe), zinc (Zn), copper (Cu), and nickel (Ni), is a heavy metal (atomic mass = 54.93) and, at the same time, a metallic micronutrient. This nutrient, similarly Fe, may be found in plant tissues at greater concentrations than necessary for appropriate functioning of the organism. Mn serves many physiological functions because it is a component of several enzymes: Mn-catalase and dehydrogenases, and it is an activator of decarboxylases, hydroxylases, acid phosphatase, and dismutase, e.g. SOD [25]. It is also found in lignins, flavonoids, and the PS II-protein complex. It plays an important role in the reactions of water splitting in the light-dependent reactions of photosynthesis. Mn is an activator of citric acid enzymes, reduction of nitrates, and metabolism of proteins, saccharides, and lipids, and it also participates in oxidation of indole-3-acetic acid (IAA) [25]. Mn indirectly controls the level of NADPH, and its extreme deficiency may cause thylakoid membrane dysfunctions. It is also involved in the tricarboxylic acid cycle, in the synthesis of chlorophyll (phosphatidic acid), and in the removal of free radicals formed in chloroplasts.

Mn is absorbed by plants as the Mn^{2+} cation, and it is passively transported through the cell membrane following the electrochemical gradient [26]. In plants, it is mainly transported in the xylem; it is sparcely reutilized; thus, the first symptoms of its deficiency are manifested in the apical parts of plants. Excessive uptake of Mn may damage the photosynthetic organs and therefore leads to reduced contents of chlorophyll and yielding of plants [27–29]. Mn tolerance of plants depends on their genome.

2.1.2. Manganese in human diet

Mn is an essential micronutrient, which has to be supplied with the diet. It plays an important role in many physiological processes, and it is required in the regulation of sugar levels, bone growth and reproduction, or proper functioning of the immune system [30]. However, there are no standards regulating the content of Mn in food. The daily allowance recommended by the National Academies' Institute of Medicine, referred to as adequate intake (AI), for this micronutrient amounts to 1.8 mg for women and 2.3 mg for men [31]. Daily intake causing no toxicity symptoms, defined as tolerable upper intake level (UL), is as high as 11 mg•day^{-1}. European nutrition standards define the optimal intake as 1–15 mg Mn•day^{-1} [32]. No symptoms of Mn deficiency are observed in free living subjects [33], and rational nutrition fully covers the daily requirement for this nutrient [34].

Vegetables are capable of accumulating this nutrient with an increase in the concentration of Mn in nutrient solution used in fertigation. The disturbed Fe/Mn ratio in food may be potentially dangerous for consumers, including vegetables more frequently consumed in season. These micronutrients compete for the same protein in blood serum (transferrin) and the protein divalent metal transporter system DMT 1 [35]. Daily uptake of Fe with food rations is sufficient for men, but very often it does not cover the safe level recommended for women [33]. In addition, it is known that the accumulation of Mn in the human organism—when the consumed diet is one of the routes of absorption of this micronutrient—may be harmful, leading to changes in the central nervous system. However, a detailed mechanism of Mn neurotoxicity is relatively little known [30,36].

2.1.3. Tomato reaction on increasing concentration of Mn in nutrient solution

This chapter shows the multifaceted response to increase Mn concentrations in nutrient solutions, ranging from insufficient to excessive/toxic: chemical changes the root zone of plants, in leaves—focusing on chosen parameters of photosynthetic activity as well as yields of fruits and their quality. It also shows a specific potential applicability of choline-stabilized orthosilicic acid (ch-OSA) in nutrient solution to alleviate Mn stress in tomato. Described studies were conducted on cultivation of two culivars: 'Alboney F_1' (*Enza Żaden*) and 'Emotion F_1' (*S&G*) grown in rockwool. In experiments, a standard nutrient solution with varying contents of Mn was used: Experiment I—control: 0.06 (native content in water), 0.3, 0.6, and 1.2 mg·dm^{-3} and Experiment II—2.4, 4.8, 9.6, and 19.2 mg·dm^{-3} [37].

2.1.3.1. Chemical composition of the root zone

The increase in Mn concentration in nutrient solution use in fertigation of tomato has a significant and multifaceted effect on the chemical composition of the rhizosphere [37]. Generally, Mn content in the root zone is significantly reduced in relation to that in nutrient solution applied in plants, but the response generally significantly varies between cultivars (**Table 1**).

Sampling place	Mn level							
	Experiment I				Experiment II			
	Mn-0	Mn-0.3	Mn-0.6	Mn-1.2	Mn-2.4	Mn-4.8	Mn-9.6	Mn-19.2
Dripper	0.06 c	0.31 e	0.57 i	1.16 j	2.45 b	4.88 e	9.78 g	19.91 j
'Alboney F_1'[1]	0.04 b	0.06 c	0.36 f	0.53 h	1.14 a	3.92 c	6.55 f	17.98 i
'Emotion F_1'[2]	0.02 a	0.14 d	0.14 d	0.42 g	1.04 a	4.40 d	10.02 g	16.66 h

Notes: Results were subjected to analysis of variance, independently for each experiment; nutrient solution collected from slabs of cv.; [1]'Alboney F_1'; [2] 'Emotion F_1'; values described with identical letters do not differ significantly at α = 0.05.

Table 1. The effect of increasing Mn concentration in nutrient solution (mg•dm^{-3}) on contents of that microelement in cultivation slabs [38].

Increasing concentrations of Mn in nutrient solution significantly modifies the chemical composition of root zone, but the reaction varies depending on cultivar and Mn concentration: in the range of Mn contents up to 1.2 mg•dm^{-3}; a significant increases: N–NO_3, Ca, Mg, S–SO_4, Zn (except for Mn-1,2), Na, and Cl; pH (alkalization) and EC, at a simultaneous reduction of contents of K (except for the control) and Fe.

2.1.3.2. *Chemical composition of leaves*

Mn nutrition and cultivar significantly influence on the chemical composition of leaves [39]. Mn content in tomato leaves is significantly connected with the contents of this nutrient in nutrient solution used in fertigation of plants and similarly in case of rhizospere generally varies between cultivars (**Table 2**).

Cultivar	Experiment I				Experiment II			
	Mn-0	Mn-0.3	Mn-0.6	Mn-1.2	Mn-2.4	Mn-4.8	Mn-9.6	Mn-19.2
			Mn content in leaves					
'Alboney F_1'	62.9 a	175.3 b	260.7 d	290.8 e	424.0 a	464.4 c	472.0 c	471.4 c
'Emotion F_1'	71.1 a	229.7 c	263.8 d	313.3 f	446.2 b	459.4 bc	465.9 c	489.5 d
			Mn content in fruits					
'Alboney F_1'	7.4 a	10.7 b	19.3 e	22.8 f	73.8 a	82.5 b	83.4 b	103.8 d
'Emotion F_1'	6.8 a	16.0 c	17.7 d	34.5 g	97.1 c	106.5 d	110.2 d	132.6 e
			Fe content in fruits					
'Alboney F_1'	94.2 e	89.7 d	85.9 cd	71.2 a	66.1 e	51.7 d	49.6 c	39.2 b
'Emotion F_1'	86.8 cd	83.1 c	76.5 b	71.4 a	57.2 d	41.3 c	37.3 b	34.6 a
			Total yield of 1 tomato plant					
'Alboney F_1'	6.05 a	6.56 c	6.32 bc	6.21 b	5.77 e	5.51 de	5.04 cde	4.44 bc

Cultivar	Experiment I				Experiment II			
	Mn-0	Mn-0.3	Mn-0.6	Mn-1.2	Mn-2.4	Mn-4.8	Mn-9.6	Mn-19.2
'Emotion F_1'	5.81 a	5.82 a	6.32 bc	5.93 a	5.42 de	4.83 cd	4.04 b	2.80 a

Notes: Results were subjected to analysis of variance, independently for each experiment; nutrient solution collected from slabs of cv.: [1]'Alboney F_1'; [2] 'Emotion F_1'; values described with identical letters do not differ significantly at α = 0.05.

Table 2. The influence of Mn nutrition on content of Mn in leaves, Fe and Mn in fruits (in mg kg^{-1} d.m.) and on total yield of 1 tomato plant (kg) [40–42].

Increasing intensity of Mn nutrition may vary the plant nutrient status in the case of Mn-0 reduces the contents of macroelements with a simultaneous increase in the contents of Fe, Zn, and Cu, whereas in the case of the Mn-1.2 combination a decrease in the contents of N, Mg, Fe, and Zn with an increase in the contents of P, K, and Ca in relation to the combination of optimal yielding [37,38,43]. Kleiber et al. [38] claimed that variation in contents of micronutrients is greater than that of macronutrients. The same authors [44] also found that the contents of trace elements (Al, Ba, Co, Cr, and Ni) in leaves of tomato grown under strong Mn stress are decreasing.

2.1.3.3. Chosen parameters of photosynthetic activity

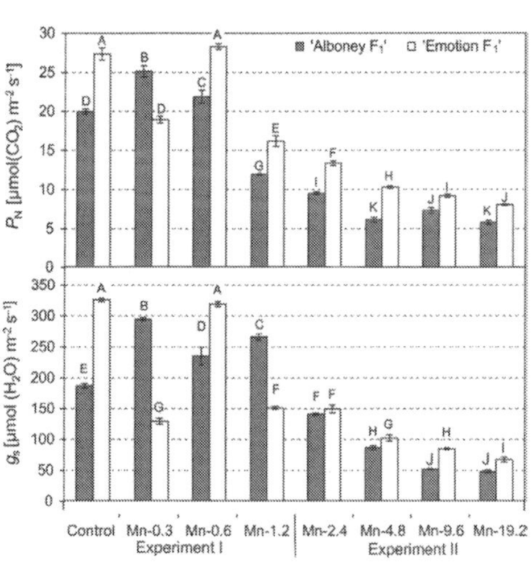

Figure 2. Means ±SE of net photosynthesis rate (PN) and stomatal conductance (gs) in tomato cultivated with different Mn in nutrient solution. Letters denote significant differences between means at p=0.05 (Kleiber et al. 2014 a).

Excessive Mn nutrition causes a toxic effect, which is observed morphologically in plants at a Mn concentration in nutrient solution ≥4.8 mg•dm^{-3} (**Figure 2**) [38, 40]; however, already at a Mn concentration of 1.2 mg•dm^{-3}, changes are observed in their photosynthetic activity. The first symptom of excessive Mn nutrition in plants is a reduction of net photosynthetic activity (P_N), although plant yielding is still visually similar to that obtained at hydroponic concentrations. With an increased intensity of Mn nutrition of plants, the values of P_N and stomatal conductance (g_s) are increasing (to 0.6 mg Mn•dm^{-3}), which indicates an adequate level of CO_2 consumption in the process of assimilation. Those parameters of photosynthetic activity significantly vary depending on the cultivar, which confirm significant variation between cultivars in relation to Mn nutrition [38].

2.1.3.4. The morphology of aboveground parts and yielding of plants

Morphological symptoms of toxic effects of Mn in the form of midrib and lateral veins browning in leaflets of a compound leaf and next necroses of compound leaves and plant apexes and inflorescence withering could be observed at the earliest after 6 weeks of culture (at Mn-19.2) and 10 weeks of exposure (at Mn-9.6) to the nutrient solution (**Figure 2**) [42,43]. For those combinations, a significant reduction in the photosynthetic activity of plants is present [38]. Symptoms of Mn deficiency on leaves could be observed earlier than toxicity—after 3 weeks (in the case of control).

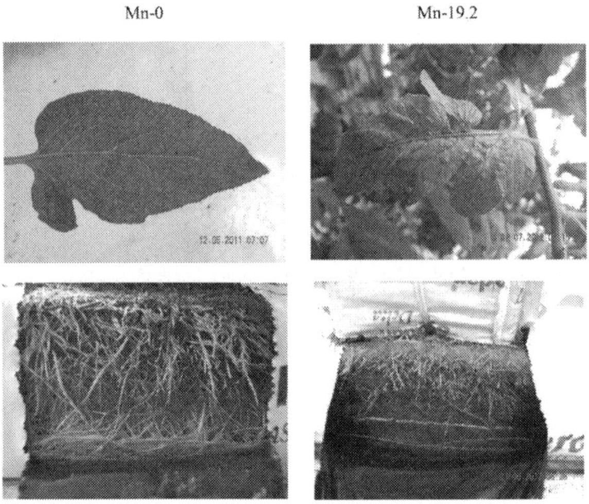

Figure 3. Morphological appearance of leaves and roots at manganese deficiency (at Mn-0) and toxicity (at Mn-19.2) Fot. Kleiber.

The hydroponic concentration of Mn for fertigation of tomato varies depending on cultivar. The greatest marketable yield of fruits in cv. 'Alboney F_1' is obtained at the Mn contents of 0.3–0.6 mg•dm^{-3} nutrient solution, but in the case of cv. 'Emotion F_1' yield for the range of maximum Mn-0.3 is lower than Mn-0.6 (**Table 2**). The content of Mn in nutrient solution amounting to 1.2 mg•dm^{-3} is excessive and contributed to a significant deterioration of yielding, at the simultaneous lack of morphological toxicity symptoms on plants. Mn stress significantly reduces not only mass of fruits but also leaves and shoots [42]. Significantly, the greatest contents of Mn are characterized leaves, whereas lowest contents are characterized fruits. There is a marked correlation between increasing contents of Mn in nutrient solutions used in fertigation of plants and its contents in leaves, stems, and fruits ($R^2 = 0.94–0.99$). A high correlation could also be observed for Mn contents between examined plant parts ($R^2 = 0.89–0.98$).

Tomato cultivars may significantly differ in relation to the requirement and tolerance to Mn concentration in nutrient solutions used in fertigation, but, generally, those species may be classified as a medium tolerance to excessive Mn concentrations in nutrient solution.

2.1.3.5. Chemical composition of fruits

Increasing intensity in Mn nutrition causes increasing in Mn concentration in fruits—but the response similarly in case of leaves generally significantly varies between cultivars (except Mn-0; Table 2) [41,44]. The range of hydroponic concentrations of Mn in fruits that are determined for cv. 'Alboney F_1' is 10.7–19.3 mg Mn•kg^{-1} d.m., whereas for cv. 'Emotion F_1,' it is 17.7 mg Mn•kg^{-1} d.m. At the greatest tested concentration of Mn for these cultivars, they are 103.8 and 132.6 mg Mn•kg^{-1} d.m. Mean Fe/Mn ratios in fruits recorded at the applied hydroponic concentrations are 1.00 : 0.15–0.22, while at the application of 19.2 mg Mn•dm^{-3}, it is 1.00 : 3.20, whereas at the nutrient solution of Mn-1.2, these ratios are 1.00 : 0.40. This indicates a marked and adverse reduction in relative Fe contents. In view of the recommended daily allowances for Mn in the human diet, it seems potentially undesirable to consume tomato fruits from plants supplied excessive or toxic levels of this nutrient.

Mn nutrition significantly impacts on the nutritive value of tomato fruits. A significant reduction is generally recorded for the contents of P, K, Ca, and Mg and the other metallic micronutrients (Fe, Zn, and Cu). Significant variation, depending on the cultivar, is shown generally for N, Ca, Mg Fe, Zn, and Cu. The greatest contents of N, Ca, and Mg in fruits are in the control, while those of P and K—at 0.3 mg Mn dm^{-3}, whereas the lowest contents of nutrients (except for N) are in the case of Mn-19.2.

The increasing intensity in Mn nutrition significantly modifies contents of trace elements (Al, Ba, Co, and Pb) in fruits, at the same time, having no effect on Cr and Cd [41]. A series of those metals in tomato fruits within the range of hydroponic concentrations of Mn are in the following: Ba 4.340–6.180 mg•kg^{-1} d.m. > Ni 4.746–5.198 mg•kg^{-1} d.m. > Co 1.014–1.064 mg•kg^{-1} d.m. > Pb 0.854–0.887 mg•kg^{-1} d.m. > Cd 0.379–0.395 mg•kg^{-1} d.m. > Cr 0.120 mg•kg^{-1} d.m. > Al 0.066–0.081 mg•kg^{-1} d.m. In the range of hydroponic Mn concentrations, contents of analyzed trace elements generally did not vary significantly between cultivars.

2.1.3.6. Use of choline-stabilized orthosilicic acid (ch-OSA) in nutrient solution to alleviate Mn stress

Studies conducted so far have indicated a significant role of silicon (Si) as an element alleviating the toxic effect of Mn [27,45–50]. Previous studies on that subject are concerned with various species, e.g. beans, barley, cucumber, rice, and cowpea. The highest Mn concentrations in nutrient solution (9.6 and 19.2 mg•dm^{-3}) cause the strongest Mn stress of tomato. One of the available forms of Si, which may be used in fertigation, is ch-OSA. Ch-OSA is also used in medicine; e.g. in combination therapy, ch-OSA/vitamin D_3 is used as a preparation affecting bone collagen in the treatment of osteoporosis [51].

The application of the tested bioavailable Si compound (ch-OSA at a scaled concentration of 0.3 mg Si•dm^{-3}) improves photosynthetic activity (**Table 3**) and results in improving plant yielding—especially for lower levels of Mn. All the factors—(i) content of Mn in nutrient solution, (ii) the application of ch-OSA, and (iii) the cultivar—significantly affect the chemical composition of leaves and tomato fruits [45,46]. Increasing in Mn stress modifies the concentration of microelements and Si in tomato leaves. Application of ch-OSA also influences the concentration of nutrients, but the determined changes were generally multidirectional and vary depending on Mn level and cultivar. Ch-OSA treatment does not influence on the Mn concentrations in fruits.

Mn level	**Ch-OSA treatment**			**Ch-OSA treatment**		
	–	+	**Mean**	–	+	**Mean**
	'Alboney F_1'			**'Emotion F_1'**		
			P_N [µmol (CO_2) m^{-2} s^{-1}]			
9.6	8.46 a	11.58 c	10.02 A	8.14 a	17.03 c	13.11 A
19.2	6.92 b	10.38 d	8.65 B	9.44 b	13.16 d	11.47 A
			g_s [µmol (H_2O) m^{-2} s^{-1}]			
9.6	80.05 b	113.83 b	96.94 A	80.26 a	151.31 c	119.00 A
19.2	69.77 a	114.40 b	92.09 A	99.50 b	122.97 d	112.31 A
			Marketable yield of 1 tomato plant			
9.6	4.88 a	5.80 b	5.35 A	4.53 b	4.89 c	4.71 B
19.2	4.78 a	4.85 a	4.80 A	4.06 a	3.85 a	3.96 A

Notes: Means in rows marked with various big letters differ significantly; means in columns marked with various big letters differ significantly; means in rows and columns marked with various small letters differ significantly.

Table 3. The influence of Mn and ch-OSA nutrition on the photosynthetic activity in leaves (P_N—net photosynthetic rate, g_s—stomatal conductance) and marketable yield of 1 tomato plant (kg) [46].

2.2. Boron

2.2.1. *Physiological role of boron*

B is an essential micronutrient for plant growth and development. It is classified as a biophilic non-metal [52]. It participates in the formation of cell–wall structures and cell divisions [53], pollen tube development [54], and saccharide metabolism [55]. Plants accumulate B through their root system [56] or through leaves [54]. B content affects nitrogen metabolism of plants, although a deficit of this micronutrient results in an increased content in nitrates in plants. Boron also plays a role in phenolic metabolism [57] and in the ascorbate–glutathione metabolic cycle [53]. It also participates in the formation and functioning of the cell wall [58]. B deficit results in the inhibition of cell–wall synthesis and affects cell elasticity [59], leading to an increase in pore size, resulting in cell–wall rupture [53]. B may form complex compounds with sugars, phenols, organic acids, and polymers [60]. Most frequently, B is found in complex combinations with mannitol, sorbitol, glucose, and fructose [60]. B may also form complex compounds with the RG-II polysaccharide [61–64] stabilized with calcium ions [53,61], the most important boron-binding compound in the cell wall. This complex is found in mono- and dicotyledonous plants [65,66].

2.2.2. *The effect of boron on human health*

The role of B in the human organism has not been fully clarified. This micronutrient determines appropriate bone development, preventing osteoporosis. An adequate B uptake with the human diet prevents arthritis [61]. B was shown to affect the activity of brain cells, the metabolism of calcium and magnesium, and the immune system [67,68]. According to Kurtoğlu et al. [69] and Li et al. [70], the interaction of B and calcium influences hormonal functions in the human. The daily dose of B absorbed by humans through the respiratory and the alimentary systems as well as the skin varies, ranging from 0.25 to 20 mg a day [71–73]. B is not accumulated in tissues, and it is excreted with urine [72], but its excess is dangerous for human health [52]. The most important sources of B in the human diet include drinks, vegetables, and fruits [74]. According to Castillo et al. [75], the greatest amounts of B are contained in beets (250 mg kg^{-1}), lemons (150 mg kg^{-1}), and apples (110 mg kg^{-1}).

2.2.3. *Boron content in water*

Natural and anthropogenic factors are sources of B in underground waters. Natural concentrations of B in fresh water result from the contents of borates in soils and rocks, mixing of waters at different aquifer levels as well as the effect of marine intrusion. During rock weathering, B penetrates to the solution forming a series of anions: BO_2^-, $B_4O_7^{-2}$, BO_3^{-3}, $H_2BO_3^-$, and $H_4BO_4^-$ [76]. Most frequently, B is found in water in the form of boric acid [77], less commonly in anions and organic compounds [71]. B content in surface and underground waters may range from 5 to 100 mg dm^{-3} [78]. Natural B content in underground waters in Poland amounts to 0.01–0.5 mg dm^{-3} [79]. According to Breś et al. [19], B content in water used in horticulture does not exceed 0.1 mg dm^{-3}; however, in areas with high intensity of horticultural production, the content of B may exceed 0.6 mg dm^{-3} [80]. Many authors [81–84] recommend an optimal B content in the nutrient solution for fertigation of tomato at 0.3 mg dm^{-3}. In studies presented by other authors, the recommended B content in the nutrient solution for tomato growing is 0.2–0.7 mg dm^{-3} [3,85–91].

2.2.4. *Material and methods*

The vegetation experiment was conducted in the years 2009–2012 (Experiment I) and 2013–2014 (Experiment II). Analyses were conducted on the effect of B fertigation on yielding and macronutrient content in leaves and fruits of tomato grown on rockwool. Vegetation experiments were run in a specialist culture greenhouse equipped with the modern climate control system. Climate parameters (such as temperature, CO_2 content, and % RH) were recorded using the Synopta software. The facilities were equipped with a modern computer-controlled fertigation system and energy-conservation curtains. Plants were grown at a density of 2.7 plants·m^{-2}.

The experiment was conducted on two tomato cv. Alboney F_1 and Emotion F_1. Plants were grown in standard rockwool (density of 60 kg·m^{-3}, mats of 100 × 15 × 7.5 cm). Experiment was established in a completely randomized system, in six replications with two plants in each. Biological pest control was applied in that culture. All cultivation measures were performed in accordance with the current recommendations for tomato growing [92]. Seeds were sown to cultivation plugs in the first half of March in each year of the study. After 2 weeks, seedlings were transplanted to rockwool cubes (10 × 10 × 10 cm). Plants were transplanted to permanent beds in the second half of April in each year of the study. The experiment was concluded on 30 September in each year of the study. The experiments were conducted in two factors (factor A—B concentration and factor B—cultivar) in five replications with four plants in each.

Plants were grown using fertigation in the closed system with no recirculation of the nutrient solution. A standard nutrient solution for tomato growing was used with the following nutrient contents: N-NH_4—2.0 mg·dm^{-3}, N-NO_3—230 mg·dm^{-3}, P—50 mg·dm^{-3}, K—420 mg·dm^{-3}, Ca—140 mg·dm^{-3}, Mg—60 mg·dm^{-3}, Cl—30 mg·dm^{-3}, S-SO_4—120 mg·dm^{-3}, Fe—1.80 mg·dm^{-3}, Mn—0.3 mg·dm^{-3}, Zn—0.50 mg·dm^{-3}, and Cu—0.07 mg·dm^{-3}. The nutrient solution of B was prepared and added individually to the respective tanks with a capacity of 1000 dm^{-3} in the following combinations: control (0.011), 0.4, 0.8, and 1.6 mg·dm^{-3} in the form of $Na_2B_4O_7 \cdot 10H_2O$ (Experiment I) and boric acid H_3BO_3 (Experiment II; combinations of the designated symbols, respectively, B-I, B-II, B-III, and B-IV). The nutrient solution dose depended on the development phase of plants and climatic conditions. In the period of intensive plant yielding and high temperatures (months June–July), 3.0–3.5 dm^3 nutrient solutions per plant were applied daily, in 15–20 single doses at 20–30% drip from mats.

In the vegetation period, the yield of fruits was recorded in terms of fruit quality grades: I—over 10.2 cm; II—10.2–8.2 cm; III—8.2–6.7 cm, IV—6.7–5.7 cm, V—5.7–4.7 cm, and VI—less than 4.7 cm. Marketable yield comprises fruits classified to Grades I–V.

Samples of nutrient solutions from the drippers and rockwool slabs representing the root zone of plants were collected at the same time of the day, using a syringe in the middle of the distance between plants, in the median axis of the slab, inserting the needle to half slab thickness, at the following dates: 15.05, 15.06, 15.07, and 16.08 of each year of the study. The average sample was collected from eight slabs. Chemical analyses of nutrient solutions were conducted directly in the tested solutions (without their stabilization) using the following methods: N-NH_4, N-NO_3—by distillation according to Bremner modified by Starck, P—colorimetrically with ammonium vanadium molybdate, K, Ca, Na—by flame photometry, Cl—nephelometrically with $AgNO_3$, S-SO_4—nephelometrically with $BaCl_2$, B—colorimetrically with curcumin; Mg, Fe, Mn, Zn, Cu—by atomic absorption spectrometry (AAS, on apparatus Carl Zeiss Jena); EC—conductometrically and pH—potentiometrically.

Leaf samples for chemical analyses were collected on 15.06, 15.07, and 16.08 in each of the years of the study. Index parts comprised 8–9 leaves counting from the top of the plant. One bulk sample was composed of 12 leaves collected from plants within a given combination. Representative samples of fruits were harvested in the second half of August in each year of the study. Collected plant material was dried at a temperature of 45–50°C and then ground. To determine total nitrogen, phosphorus, potassium, calcium, and magnesium contents, plant material was mineralized in concentrated sulfuric acid. Nutrient contents were determined using the following methods: N—total—by the distillation method according to Kjeldahl in a Parnas–Wagner apparatus, P—by colorimetry with ammonium molybdate (according to Schillak), while K, Ca, and Mg—by atomic absorption spectrometry (AAS). To determine total contents of iron, manganese, zinc, and copper, the plant material was mineralized in a mixture of acetic and perchloric acids (3:1 v/v), B—dry mineralization with calcium oxide (CaO). After mineralization, Fe, Mn, Zn, and Cu were determined according to AAS and B colorimetrical-ly with curcum.

Results of biometric measurements and laboratory analyses were analyzed statistically using the Duncan test, with inference at $\alpha = 0.05$.

2.2.5. *Results and discussion*

2.2.5.1. *Yielding*

The effect of B fertigation on the marketable yield of tomato fruit was found in a vegetation experiment conducted in the years 2009–2012 (Experiment I) and 2013–2014 (Experiment II; Table 4). The mean marketable yield differed significantly depending on the level of B in the nutrient solution. The largest yield marketable varieties Alboney F1 (Experiment I) obtained in combinations of B-I and B-II (5.55 and 5.52 kg · plant^{-1}). Increasing the B content of the medium had a significant effect on reducing the commercial yield in combinations of B-III and B-IV (5.09 and 5.18 kg · plant^{-1}) when compared to combinations of B-I and B-II. The highest yield of marketable varieties obtained Emotion F1 in combination of B-II (5.57 kg plant^{-1}). There were no significant differences in yield trading between combinations of B-I, B-III, and B-IV, average marketable yield of these varieties did not differ significantly. In the conducted in the years 2013 – 2014 found the experience of growing influence of fertigation boron on the marketable yield of tomato fruit. The resulting average yield commercial differ significantly depending on the level of B in the medium. In the performed experiment, no significant changes were found in the shares of the marketable yield in the total yield (99.6–100.0%). When analyzing the produced marketable yield, it needs to be stressed that the optimal level of B in the nutrient solution for cv. Alboney F_1 amounts to 0.011–0.40 mg dm^{-3}, whereas for cv. Emotion F_1 0.40 mg B · dm^{-3}. Increased B content in the nutrient solution caused a significant reduction of the marketable yield in both cultivars. Cultivar Emotion F_1 responded with a decrease in the marketable yield both to a deficit and excess B in the nutrient solution. Recorded results indicate a greater optimal content range in cv. Alboney F_1 for this micronutrient in the nutrient solution used in fertigation. In this study, when applying a nutrient solution consid-ered to be standard (0.40 mg dm^{-3}), a similar marketable yield was found for cv. Emotion F_1

(5.85 kg plant^{-1}) to that obtained by Kleiber [43] when using a standard nutrient solution (5.82 kg plant^{-1}). No differences were observed between cultivars, and the produced marketable yield of cv. Alboney F_1 was lower by ±0.7 kg plant^{-1}. The effect of B on yielding in tomato was confirmed by a study conducted by Oyinlola [93]. In comparison with the experiment carried out by Piróg and Komosa [94], the produced marketable yield in both cultivars in this experiment at B contents in the nutrient solution of 0.0, 0.4, and 0.8 mg dm^{-3} was greater, it may have a significant effect at mass-scale tomato production. In an experiment conducted by Jarosz and Dzida [81], the greatest total yield of cv. 'Cunero F1' was 14.7 kg m^{-2} (2.7 plant m^{-2}), whereas studies carried out in 2004 on the same cultivar showed a yield of 4.39 kg plant^{-1} [9].

Variety	B-I	B-II	B-III	B-IV	Mean
		Experiment I			
		Marketable field (kg plant^{-1})			
Alboney F_1	5.55 c	5.52 c	5.09 ab	5.18 b	5.34 A
Emotion F_1	5.00 a	5.57 c	4.92 a	4.74 a	5.06 A
Średnia Mean	5.28 AB	5.55 B	5.01 A	4.96 A	
		Contribution of marketable yield in total yield (%)			
Alboney F_1	99.5	99.5	99.2	99.4	99.4
Emotion F_1	99.6	99.1	99.2	99.4	99.3
Średnia Mean	99.6	99.3	99.2	99,4	
		Experiment II			
		Marketable field (kg plant^{-1})			
Alboney F_1	5.73 bc	5.87 c	5.65 b	5.46 a	5.68 A
Emotion F_1	5.24 a	5.85 c	5.60 b	5.41 a	5.52 A
Mean	5.48 A	5.86 C	5.63 B	5.43 A	
		Contribution of marketable yield in total yield (%)			
Alboney F_1	99.8	100.0	99.8	99.6	99.8
Emotion F_1	99.8	99.7	99.8	99.6	99.7
Mean	99.8	99.8	99.8	99.6	

Notes: Means in rows marked with various big letters differ significantly; means in columns marked with various big letters differ significantly; means in rows and columns marked with various small letters differ significantly.

Table 4. The influence of B nutrition on total yield of 1 tomato plant (kg).

2.2.5.2. *Chemical composition of the root zone*

The effect of increasing B concentrations in nutrient solutions is shown (**Table 5**). In all the combinations, an increase was shown for B contents in nutrient solutions absorbed from mats in comparison with the nutrient solution applied to plants. The greatest B content in nutrient solutions for both cultivars was recorded in mats applying B at 1.60 mg dm^{-3}. Differences between cultivars were shown in terms of B content in nutrient solutions collected from mats in combinations of B-I and B-IV (Experiment I) and B-II and B-IV (Experiment II). An increase in B content in the nutrient solution in combinations of B-III and B-IV caused a significant decrease in the marketable yield, which may have been caused by the toxic individual effect of this ion on plants [95]. In this experiment, the phenomenon of B condensation was observed in growing mats, confirming the results reported by other authors [24]. It needs to be stated that B content in growing mats exceeding 0.93 mg dm^{-3} (Experiment I) causes a significant reduction of plant yielding. However, a further increase in the content of B in nutrient solutions in the rhizosphere up to 1.87 mg dm^{-3} does not cause a significant reduction of the marketable yield between these combinations. The conducted Experiment II using boric acid as a source of B in the nutrient solution showed identical dependencies in the case of the greatest marketable yield; however, the content of B in mats close to 2.00 mg dm^{-3} caused a significant reduction of yielding in comparison with combination of B-III (±1.00 mg·dm^{-3}). The highest marketable yield varieties Emotion F1 obtained when the boron content of mats 0.58 (Experiment I) and 0.67 mg·dm^{-3} (Experiment II). At the application of the same B levels in hydroponic culture of butter lettuce, a yield-modifying effect of increasing B concentrations in the nutrient solution was found for the mean weight of lettuce heads. The greatest weight of lettuce heads was produced using B content in the nutrient solution within the range of 0.40–1.60 mg dm^{-3} [96].

Sampling place	B-I	B-II	B-III	B-IV	B-I	B-II	B-III	B-IV
	Experiment I				Experiment II			
Dripper	0.11 a	0.41 d	0.80 f	1.57 h	0.11 a	0.41 c	0.82 f	1.63 h
Alboney	0.21 b	0.58 e	0.93 g	1.87 i	0.27 b	0.59 d	0.99 g	1.92 i
Emotion	0.26 c	0.58 e	0.96 g	2.00 j	0.32 b	0.67 e	1.01 g	2.11 j

Notes: Results were subjected to analysis of variance, independently for each experiment; nutrient solution collected from slabs of cv.: [1]'Alboney F_1'; [2] 'Emotion F_1'; values described with identical letters do not differ significantly at α = 0.05.

Table 5. The effect of increasing B concentration in nutrient solution (mg•dm^{-3}) on contents of that microelement in cultivation slabs.

2.2.5.3. *Chemical composition of leaves*

An increase in B contents in the nutrient solution applied in fertigation had a significant effect on the content of this micronutrient in indicator parts of tomato (**Table 6**). In combinations of B-II and B-III, an increase in B contents in the nutrient solution caused an increase in B content by ±100%. Significantly, the greatest mean B content was assayed using the nutrient solution of 1.60 (207.07 mg·kg^{-1}). Significant differences in the mean B content in leaves were observed between cultivars. According to the studies conducted by other authors, an increase in the content of B in the nutrient solution has a significant effect on contents of this micronutrient in tomato leaves [93]. [79] when growing tomato at a toxic level of boron in the nutrient solution assayed 155 mg B·kg^{-1} in tomato leaves. Results in this study for B contents in indicator parts of tomato at 0.80 and 1.60 indicate a toxic state of nutrition of plants in the case of the investigated micronutrient. According to Kabata-Pendias and Pendias [71], an admissible B content for tomato plants is 100 mg·kg^{-1} B in d.m. In turn, according to De Kreij et al. [97], an optimal content of B in tomato leaves should be 54.0–75.6 mg·kg^{-1} B d.m. When analyzing the state of nutrition of plants in the case of boron, we need to state that in this study (Experiment I) plants of cv. Alboney F_1 yielded best at B contents in indicator parts of 33.24–78.58 mg·kg^{-1}, whereas for cv. Emotion F_1 it was at 79.44 mg·kg^{-1}. In analyses with the use of boric acid (Experiment II), cv. Alboney F_1 yielded best at B contents in indicator parts of 32.80–80.62 mg·kg^{-1}, whereas for cv. Emotion F_1 at 83.89 mg·kg^{-1}. Recorded B contents were lower than those reported by Komosa et al. [23] in their studies on yielding of cv. Emotion F_1 in closed systems with recirculation and without recirculation of the nutrient solution.

Variety	B-I	B-II	B-III	B-IV	Mean
		Experiment I			
		B content in leaves			
Alboney F_1	33.24 a	78.58 b	167.46 d	207.02 f	121.57 B
Emotion F_1	37.94 a	79.44 b	139.83 c	188.68 e	111.47 A
Mean	35.59 A	79.01 B	153.65 C	197.85 D	
		Experiment II			
		B content in leaves			
Alboney F_1	32.80 a	80.62 c	173.56 e	218.30 g	126.32 B
Emotion F_1	45.17 b	83.89 c	148.61 d	195.83 f	118.37 A
Mean	38.98 A	82.25 B	161.09 C	207.07 D	

Notes: Means in rows marked with various big letters differ significantly; means in columns marked with various big letters differ significantly; means in rows and columns marked with various small letters differ significantly.

Table 6. The influence of boron nutrition on content of B in leaves (in mg kg^{-1} d.m.).

2.2.5.4. *Chemical composition of fruits*

In this study, the content of B in tomato fruits was dependent on B content in the nutrient solution used in fertigation (**Table 7**). The greatest B content in fruits of tomato cv. Alboney F_1 was recorded in combinations B-III (16.30 mg·kg^{-1}) and B-IV (16.43 mg·kg^{-1}), while for cv. Emotion F_1 in combination B-IV (17.30 mg·kg^{-1}). Differences in B contents in fruits were shown only in the B-II combination (Experiment I). In all the combinations, significant differences were observed between cultivars in terms of B contents (Experiment II). Significantly greater B contents were assayed in fruits of cv. Emotion F_1. The greatest mean B content in fruits was recorded in combination B-IV (26.50 mg·kg^{-1}). According to other authors, the content of B in tomato fruits is significantly lower in comparison with those recorded in leaves [98,99]. Results obtained in studies on the application of borax for B contents in fruits were lower than those

http://dx.doi.org/10.5772/62263

reported by Komosa et al. [24]. Using boric acid, greater boron levels were found in fruits, while differences were found between cultivars in the mean B content in tomato fruits.

Variety	B-I	B-II	B-III	B-IV	Mean
		Experiment I			
		B content in fruits			
Alboney F_1	11.66 a	13.10 b	16.30 de	16.43 de	14.60 A
Emotion F_1	11.56 a	14.26 c	15.30 cd	17.30 e	14.37 A
Mean	11.61 A	13.68 B	15.80 C	16,86 D	
		Experiment II			
		B content in fruits			
Alboney F_1	11.66 a	16.70 b	19.90 c	24.26 d	18.13 A
Emotion F_1	15.33 b	19.56 c	24.10 d	28.73 e	21.93 B
Mean	13.49 A	18.31 B	22.00 C	26.50 D	

Notes: Means in rows marked with various big letters differ significantly; means in columns marked with various big letters differ significantly; means in rows and columns marked with various small letters differ significantly.

Table 7. The influence of boron nutrition on content of B in fruits (in mg kg^{-1} d.m.).

3. Conclusions

1. When analyzing the produced marketable yield, it needs to be stressed that the optimal level of B in the nutrient solution for cv. Alboney F_1 amounts to 0.011–0.40 mg dm^{-3}, while for cv. Emotion F_1 0.40 mg B dm^{-3}. Increased B content in the nutrient solution caused a significant reduction of the marketable yield in both cultivars. Cultivar Emotion F_1 responded with a decrease in the marketable yield both to a deficit and excess B in the nutrient solution.

2. It needs to be stated that B content in growing mats exceeding 0.93 mg dm^{-3} (Experiment I) causes a significant reduction of plant yielding. However, a further increase in the content of B in nutrient solutions in the rhizosphere up to 1.87 mg dm^{-3} does not cause a significant reduction of the marketable yield between these combinations. The conducted Experiment II using boric acid as a source of B in the nutrient solution showed identical dependencies in the case of the greatest marketable yield; however, the content of B in mats close to 2.00 mg dm^{-3} caused a significant reduction of yielding in comparison with combination B-III (±1.00 mg·dm^{-3}).

3. An increase in B contents in the nutrient solution applied in fertigation had a significant effect on the content of this micronutrient in indicator parts of tomato. Results in this study for B contents in indicator parts of tomato at 0.80 and 1.60 indicate a toxic state of nutrition of plants in the case of the investigated micronutrient.

4. In this study, the content of B in tomato fruits was dependent on B content in the nutrient solution used in fertigation. Using boric acid, greater boron levels were found in fruits, while differences were found between cultivars in the mean B content in tomato fruits.

Author details

Bartosz Markiewicz, Tomasz Kleiber and Maciej Bosiacki

Department of Plant Nutrition, University of Life Sciences, Poznan, Poland

References

[1] Piróg J. Growing plants in greenhouses on various substrates. National sympodium. Poznań; 1994. (In Polish).

[2] Komosa A. Inert media – progress or inertia?. Advances of Agricultural Sciences Problem 2002: 485 147–167. (In Polish).

[3] Komosa A., Kleiber T., Markiewicz B. The effect of nutrient solutions on yield and macronutrient status of greenhouse tomato (*Lycopersicon esculentum* Mill.) grown in aeroponic and rockwool culture with or without recirculation of nutrient solution. Acta Sci. Pol. Hortorum. Cultus 2014; 13 (2), 163–177.

[4] Pudelski T. Tomatoes under glass and foil. Warszawa: PWRiL; 1998. (In Polish).

[5] Kleiber T., Markiewicz B., Niewiadomska A. Organic substrates for intensive horticultural cultures: Yield and nutrient status of plants, microbiological parameters of substrates. Pol. J. Environ. Stud. 2012; 21 (5), 1261–1271.

[6] Pawlińska A., Komosa A. The effect of substrates and nutrient solutions on yield of greenhouse tomato. Rocz. AR Pozn. CCCL VI Ogrodn. 2004; 37, 173–180 (in Polish).

[7] ANTHURA. Cultivation Guide Anthurium. Anthura; 1998, 43.

[8] Jarosz Z., Horodko K. The yielding and mineral composition of greenhouse tomato grown in inert media. Rocz. AR Pozn. CCCLIV Ogrodn. 2004; 37, 81–86.

[9] Jarosz Z., Horodko K. The yielding and mineral composition of greenhouse tomato grown in inert media. Rocz. AR Pozn. CCCLIV Ogrodn. 2004; 37, 81– 86.

[10] RuniaW.TH., Amsing JJ. Disinfection of recirculation water from closed cultivation systems by heat treatment. Acta Hort. 2001; 548, 215–222.

[11] Van Os EA. Heat treatment for disinfecting draincoater technological and economic aspects. Proc. 7th Int. Congr. Soilless Culture, Flevohof, 1988, 353–359.

[12] Van Os EA. New developments in recircualtion systems and disinfection methods for greenhouse crops. Hort. Eng. 2001; 16 (2), 2–5.

[13] Wohlanka W. Water disinfection. Taspo Praxis 1990; 18, 73–81.

[14] Benoit F., Ceustermans N. Horticultural aspects ecobiological soilless growing methods. Acta Hort. 1995; 396, 11–19.

[15] Runia WTH., Amsing JJ. Disinfestation of nematode infested recirculation water by ozone and activated hydrogen peroxide. Proceedings of 9th International Congress on Soilless Culture, St. Helier, Jersey, 12–19 April 1996.

[16] Nurzyński J. Fertilization of horticultural plants. Lublin: Wyd. AR; 2003, 1–153 (in Polish).

[17] Baran S. Possibilities of the use of GRODAN mineral wool to form water properties insoils and grounds. Advances of Agricultural Sciences Problem 2008; 535, 15 (in Polish).

[18] Dubsky M., Šramek F. The effect of rockwool on physical properties of growing substrates for perennial. Hort. Sci. (Prague) 2009; 36 (1), 38.

[19] Breś W., Kleiber T., Trelka T. Quality of water used for drip irrigation and fertigation of horticultural plants. Folia Hort. 2010; 22 (2), 67–74.

[20] Kleiber T. Pollution of the natural environment in intensive cultures under greenhouses. Archiv. Environ. Protect. 2012; 38 (2), 45–53.

[21] Gajc-Wolska J., Bujalski D., Chrzanowska A. Effect of substrate on yielding and quality of greenhouse cucumber fruits. J. Elementol. 2008; 13 (2), 205–210.

[22] Komosa A., Piróg J., Kleiber T. Changes of macro and micronutrients in the root environment of greenhouse tomato grown in fiber wood. Veg. Crps. Res. Bull. 2009; 70, 71–80.

[23] Komosa A., Kleiber T., Piróg J. Contents of macro- and microelements in root environment of greenhouse tomato grown in rockwool and wood fiber depending on nitrogen levels in nutrient solutions. Acta Sci. Pol. Hortorum. Cultus 2010; 9 (3), 59–68.

[24] Komosa A.,Piróg J., Weber Z., Markiewicz B. Comparison of yield, nutrient solution changes and nutritional status of greenhouse tomato (*Lycopersicon esculentum* Mill.) grown in recirculating and non-recirculating nutrient solution systems. J. Plant Nutr. 2011; 34, 1473–1488. DOI:10.1080/01904167.2011.585204.

[25] Kozłowska M., Bandurska H., Floryszak-Wieczorek J., Politycka B. Plant physiology PWRiL; 2007. (In Polish).

[26] Kozik E., Komosa A. The influence of macro- and micronutrients on yield quantity and quality.In: Komosa A., Breś W., Golcz A., Kozik E. (Red.), Horticultural plants nutrition. Fundamentals and prospects. PWRiL; 2012, 204–205. (In Polish).

[27] Maksimović DJ., Bogdanović J., Maksimović V., Nikolić M. Silicon modulates the metabolism and utilization of phenolic compounds in cucumber (*Cucumis sativus* L.) grown at excess manganese. J. Plant Nutr. Soil Sci. 2007; 170, 739–744.

[28] Savvas D., Papastavrou D., Ntatsi G., Ropokis A., Olympios C. Interactive effects of grafting and manganese supply on growth, yield, and nutrient uptake by tomato. HortScience 2009; 44 (7), 1978–1982.

[29] Shenker M., Plessner OE., Tel-Or E. Manganese nutrition effects on tomato growth, chlorophyll concentration, and superoxide dismutase activity. J. Plant Physiol. 2004; 161, 197–202.

[30] Aschner JL., Aschner M. Nutritional aspects of manganese homeostasis. Mol. Aspects Med. 2005; 26 (4), 353–362.

[31] Dri. Dietary references intakes for vitamin A, vitamin K, arsenic, boron, chromium, copper, iodine, iron, manganese, molybdenum, nickel, silicon, vanadium and zinc. 2002. www.nap.edu/books/0309072794/html.

[32] Nutrition Working Group of International Life Sciences Institute Europe. Recommended daily amounts of vitamins and minerals in Europe. Nutr. Abstracts Rev. A 1990; 60, 827–842.

[33] Marzec Z., Marzec A., Zaręba S. Survive daily food rations source of iron and manganese 16 for adults. Roczniki PZH. 2004, 29–34. (In Polish).

[34] Kłos A., Bertrandt J., Stężycka E., Szymańska W. Copper, zinc, magnesium and manganese content in daily food rations used for alimentation of students of the main school of fire service in Warsaw. Bromat. Chem. Toksykol. 2011; XLIV (3), 336–340 (in Polish).

[35] Roth AJ., Garrick MD. Iron interactions and biological interactions mediating the physiological ant toxic actions of manganese. Biochem. Pharmocol. 2003; 66, 1–13.

[36] Dobson AW., Erikson KM., Aschner M. Manganese neurotoxicity. Ann. N.Y. Acad. Sci. 2004; 1012, 115–128.

[37] Kleiber T. Studies on increasing manganese nutrition effect of tomato (*Lycopersicon esculentum* Mill.) on differentiation of rhizosphere chemical composition. Scientific and Didactic Equipment 2014a; 2, 119–126.

[38] Kleiber T., Borowiak K., Budka A., Kayzer D. Relations between Mn concentration and yield, nutrient, water status, and gas exchange parameters of tomato. Acta Biol. Cracoviens. Series Bot. 2014a; 56 (2), 98–106.

[39] Kleiber T. Effect of manganese on nutrient content in tomato (*Lycopersicon esculentum* Mill.) leaves. J. Elementol. 2015; 20 (1), 115–126. DOI:10.5601/jelem.2014.19.2.580.

[40] Kleiber T., Szablewski T., Stuper-Szablewska K., Cegielska-Radziejewska R. Determination of correlations between content of manganese in nutrient solution and concentration of trace elements in tomato fruits (*Lycopersicon esculentum* Mill.). Food. Science. Technology. Quality 2014b; 6 (97), 81–91 (in Polish).

[41] Kleiber T., Szablewski T., Stuper-Szablewska K., Cegielska-Radziejewska R. Determination of manganese stress influence on content of trace elements in leaves of

tomatoes (*Lycopersicon esculentum* Mill.) Bromat. Chem. Toksykol. 2014c; XLVII (I), 89–95 (in Polish).

[42] Kleiber T., Grajek M. Tomato reaction on excessive manganese nutrition. Bulgarian J. Agric. Sci. 2015; 21 (1), 124–131.

[43] Kleiber T. Influence of manganese on yielding of tomato (*Lycopersicon esculentum* Mill.) cultivated in rockwool. Nauka Przyroda Technol. 2014b; 8 (2), 14.

[44] Kleiber T. Changes of nutrient contents in tomato fruits under the influence of increasing intensity of manganese nutrition. Ecol. Chem. Eng. S 2014c; 21 (2), 297–307.

[45] Kleiber T., Bosiacki M., Breś W. The effect of ch-OSA application on tomato grown under increasing manganese stress. J. Elementol. 2015a; 20 (4), 897–910. DOI:10.5601/jelem. 2015.20.1.820.

[46] Kleiber T., Calomme M., Borowiak K. The effect of choline-stabilized orthosilicic acid on microelements and silicon concentration, photosynthesis activity and yield of tomato grown under Mn stress. Plant Physiol. Biochem. 2015b; 96, 180–188.

[47] Horiguchi T. Mechanism of manganese toxicity and tolerance of plants IV. Effects of silicon on alleviation of manganese toxicity of rice plants. Soil Sci. Plant Nutr. 1988; 34 (1), 65–73.

[48] Iwasaki K., Maier P., Fecht M., Horst WJ. Effects of silicon supply on apoplastic manganese concentrations in leaves and their relation to manganese tolerance in cowpea (*Vigna unguiculata* (L.) Walp.). Plant Soil 2002; 238, 281–288.

[49] Liang Y., Wanchun S., Yong-Guan Z., Christie P. Mechanisms of silicon-mediated alleviation of abiotic stresses in higher plants: A review. Environ. Pollut. 2007; 147 (2), 422–428.

[50] Zanão Júnior LA., Ferreira Fontes RL., Lima Neves JC., Korndörfer GH., Vinícius Tavares de Ávila V. Rice grown in nutrient solution with doses of manganese and silicon. R. Bras. Ci Solo. 2010; 34, 1629–1639.

[51] Spector TD., Calomme MR., Anderson SH., Clement G., Bevan L., Demeester N., Swaminathan R., Jugdaohsingh R., Vanden Berghe DA., Powell JJ. Choline-stabilized orthosilicic acid supplementation as an adjunct to calcium/vitamin D3 stimulates markers of bone formation in osteopenic females: A randomized, placebo-controlled trial. BMC Musculoskelet. Disord. 2008; 9, 85.

[52] Tomaszewska B. Boron in groundwater and landfill leachate. Exploration Technology Geothermal Energy, Sustainable development nr 1–2/2010. 161 – 171.

[53] Brown P.H., Bellalui N., Wimmer M.A., Bassil E.S., Ruiz J., Hu H., Pffefer H., Dannel F., Romheld V. (2002): Boron in plant biology. Plant Biology 4/2: 205 – 223.

[54] Lityński T., Jurkowska H. Soil fertility and plant nutrition. Warszawa: PWN; 1982. (In Polish).

[55] Shol'nik MY. The Physiological Role of B in Plants. London, UK: Borax Consolidated Limited; 1965.

[56] Fotyma M., Mercik S. Agricultural Chemistry II. Warszawa: Wyd PWN; 1995 (in Polish).

[57] Ruiz JM., Bretones G., Baghour M., Ragala L., Belakbir A., Romero L. Relationship between boron and phenolic metabolism in tobacco leaves. Phytochemistry 1998b; 48, 269–272.

[58] O'Neill MA., Ishii T., Albersheim P., Darvill AG. Rhamnogalacturonan II: Structure and function of a borate cross-linked cell wall pectic polysaccharide. Annu. Rev. Plant Biol. 2004; 55, 109–139.

[59] Biernat J., Pieczyńska J. The role of boron in the metabolism and in human nutrition. Bromatologia chemistry and toxicology. 2000; 33 (4), 289–294. (In Polish).

[60] Hu H., Brown PH. Localisation of boron in cell walls ofsquash and tobacco and its association with pectin. Plant Physiol. 1994; 105, 681–689.

[61] Goldbach HE., Rerkasem B., Wimmer MA., Brown PH., Thellier M., Bell RW. Boron in Plant and Animals Nutrition. New York: Kluwer Academic/Plenum Publishers; 2002.

[62] Kobayashi M., Matoh T., Azuma J. Two chains of rhamnogalacturonan II are cross-linked by borate-diol ester bonds in higher plant cell walls. Plant Physiol. 1996; 110, 1017–1020.

[63] O'Neill MA. Warrenfeltz D, Kates K, Pellerin P Doco T Darvill AG, Albersheim P. Rhamnogalacturona – II, a pectic polysaccharide in the walls of growing plant cell, forms a dimer that is covalently cross-linked by a borate ester – In vitro conditions for the formation and hydrolysis of the dimer. J. Biol. Chem. 1996; 271,22923–22930.

[64] O'Neill MA., Eberhard S., Albersheim P., Darvill AG. Requirement of borate cross-linking of cell wall rhamnogalacturonan II for *Arabidopsis* growth. Science 2001; 294, 846–849.

[65] Ishii T., Matsunaga T., Hayashi N. Formation of rhamnogalacturonan II-borate dimer in pectin determines cell wall thickness of pumpkin tissue. Plant Physiol. 2001; 126, 1698–1705.

[66] Kaneko S., Ishii T., Matsunaga T. A boron-rhamngalcturonan-II complex from bamboo shoot cell walls. Phytochemistry 1997; 44, 243–248.

[67] Murray F.J. A human health risk assessment of boron (boric acid and borax) in drinking water. Regul. Toxicol. Pharmacol. 1995; 22 (3), 221–230.

[68] Nielsen F.H. The emergence of boron as nutritionally import ant throughout the life cycle. Nutrition 2000; 16, 512–514.

[69] Kurtoğlu V., Kurtoğlu F., Coşkun B. Effects of boron supplementation of adequate and inadequate vitamin D_3-containing diet on performance and serum biochemical characters of broiler chickens. Res. Vet. Sci. 2001; 71, 183–187.

[70] Li Q., Zhang T. A novel method of the determination of boron in the presence of a little metanol by discoloring spectrophotometry in pharmaceutitcal an biological samales. Talanta 2007; 71, 296–302.

[71] Kabata-Pendias A., Pendias H. Biogeochemistry of trace elements. Warszawa: Wyd. Nauk, PWN; 1999. (In Polish).

[72] Moore JA., Expert Scientific Committee. An assessment of boric acid and borax using the IEHR evaluative process for assessing human developmental and reproductive toxicity of agents. Reprod. Toxicol. 1997; 11 (1), 123–160.

[73] Rainey CJ., Nyquist LA., Christensen RE. Daily boron intake from the American diet. J. Am. Dietet. Assoc. 1998; 99, 335–340.

[74] Biego GH., Joyeux M., Hartemann P., Derby G. Daily intake of essentials minerals and metalic micropollutants from foods in France. Sci. Total Environ. 1998; 217, 27–36.

[75] Castillo J.R., Mir J.M., Bendicho C., Martinez C. Determination of boron in waters by using methyl borate generation and flame atomic-emission spektrometry. Atomic Spectroscopy. 1985. 6. 152 – 155.

[76] Kabata-Pendias A., Pendias H. Trace Elements in Soli and Plants. Boca-Raton, FL: CRC Press; 2001.

[77] ItakuraT., SasaiR., ItohH. Precipitation recovery of boron from wastewater by hydrothermal mineralization. Water Res. 2005; 39 (12), 2543–2548.

[78] Melnyk L., Goncharuk V., Butnyk I., Eugene Tsapiuk E. Boron removal from natural and wastewaters using combined sorption/membrane process. Desalination 2005; 185, 147–157.

[79] RMS. J. Laws 2008; 143, item 896.

[80] Kowalczyk W., Dyśko J., Felczyńska A. Evaluation of the nutrient elements polution level of the groundwater intakes on the concentrated areas of greenhouse production. Vegetable News. 2010.51. 29 – 34. (In Polish).

[81] Jarosz Z., Dzida K. Effect of substratum and nutrient solution upon yielding and chemical composition of leaves and fruits of glasshouse tomato grown in prolonged cycle. Acta Sci. Pol. Hortorum. Cultus 2011; 10 (3), 247–258.

[82] Jarosz Z., Dzida K., Nurzyńska-Wierdak R. Possibility of reusing expanded clay in greenhouse tomato cultivation. Part i. Yield and chemical composition of fruits. Acta Sci. Pol. Hortorum Cultus 2012; 11 (6), 119–130.

[83] Kowalczyk K., Gajc-Wolska J. Effect of the kind of growing medium and transplant grafting on the cherry tomato yielding. Acta Sci. Pol. Hortorum Cultus 2011; 10 (1), 61–70.

[84] Wysocka-Owczarek M. Tomatoes under Cover. The Cultivation of Conventional and Modern. Warszawa: Hortpress Sp. z o.o; 1998, 166–187 (in Polish).

[85] Adams P., Nutrition of greenhouse vegetables in NFT and hydroponics systems. Acta Hort. 1994; 361, 245–257.

[86] Borowski E., Nurzyński J. Effect of different growing substrates on the photosynthesis parameters and fruit yield of greenhouse-grown tomato. Acta Sci. Pol. Hortorum. Cultus 2012; 11 (6), 95–105.

[87] Hochmuth GJ., Hochmuth RC. Nutrient Solution Formulation for Hydroponic (Perlite, Rockwool, NFT) Tomatoes. Florida: University of Florida, HS796; 2012.

[88] Kleiber T., Markiewicz B. Application of 'Tytanit' in grenhouse tomato growning. Acta Sci. Pol. Hortorum. Cultus 2013; 12 (3), 117–126.

[89] Komosa A., Górniak T. The effect of chloride on nutrie nt contents in fruits of greenhouse tomato (*Lycopersicon esculentum* Mill.) Grown in rockwool. Acta Sci. Pol. Hortorum. Cultus 2012; 11 (5), 43–53.

[90] Markiewicz B., Kleiber T. The effect of Tytanit application on the content of selected microelements and the biological value of tomato fruits. J. Elem. 2014; 19 (4), 1065–1072. DOI:10.5601/jelem.2014.19.3.486.

[91] Zekki H., Gauthier L., Gosselin A. Growth, productivity and mineral composition of hydroponically cultivated greenhouse tomatoes, with or without nutrient solution recycling. J. Am. Soc. Hort. Sci. 1996; 121 (6), 1082–1088.

[92] Adamicki F., Dyśko J., Nawrocka B., Ślusarski C., Wysocka-Owczarek M. Methodology of Integrated Production of Tomatoes under Cover. Warszawa: PIORIN; 2005 (in Polish).

[93] Oyinlola EY. Distribution of boron and its uptake in the plants parts of two tomato varietes. Chem. Class J. 2005; 2, 77–80.

[94] Piróg J., Komosa A. Influence of substrate and cultivar on quantity and quality of greenhouse tomato yield. Acta Agrophys. 2006; 7 (3), 699–707 (in Polish).

[95] Breś W., Golcz A., Komosa A., Kozik E., Tyksiński W. Horticulture plant nutrition. Wydawnictwo UP; 2009. Poznań. (In Polish).

[96] Markiewicz B., Bosiacki M., Kleiber T. Effect of boron fertigation on yield and nutrientcontent of lettuce grown (*Lactuca sativa* L.) in the closed fertigation system with recirculation of the nutrient solution. ABiD 2013; 4: 318 – 322, 2013.

[97] De KreijC., SonneveldC., WarmenhovenM.G., StraverN. Guide values for nutrient element contents of vegetables and flowers under glass. Voedingsoplossingen Glastuinbouw 1990; 23.

[98] Garate A.J., Carpena-Ruiz R.O., Ramon A.M. Influence of boron on manganese and other nutrients in tissues sets of conductors . Annals of Soil Science and Agricultural Biology1984, 43: 1467–1477.

[99] Gupta UC. Boron nutrition of crops. Adv. Agron. 1979; 31, 273–305.

[100] Roth AJ., Garrick MD. Iron interactions and biological interactions mediating the physiological ant toxic actions of manganese. Biochem. Pharmocol. 2003; 66, 1–13.

[101] TomaszewskaB. Boron in Groundwater and Waste Dump Leachates. Technika Poszukiwań Geologicznych Geotermia, Zrównoważony Rozwój; 2010, 161–171 (in Polish).

Chapter 7

Analysis of Soil Profile Water Storage under Sunflower × Cowpea Intercrop in the Limpopo Province of South Africa

Jestinos Mzezewa and Eastonce T. Gwata

Additional information is available at the end of the chapter

http://dx.doi.org/10.5772/62764

Abstract

Sunflower (*Helianthus annuus* L.) is the most important oilseed crop in South Africa. Its production in semi-arid area is limited by low rainfall exacerbated by high temperatures that deplete soil moisture. Cowpea (*Vigna unguiculta*) intercropped in sunflower could reduce evaporation of soil moisture by increasing soil cover. A field study was carried out 2007/2008 and 2008/2009 seasons in the Limpopo Province (South Africa) to compare (i) the changes in soil profile water storage, (ii) water use efficiency, and (iii) productivity of the sunflower–cowpea cropping systems. Extraction patterns by layers showed no significant differences in all cropping systems in the 0–300, 300–600, and 600–900 mm during 2007/2008 and 2008/2009 seasons. Sole sunflower (SS) significantly extracted more soil water than sole cowpea and the intercrop from the 1200- to 1500-mm layer after 56 days after planting (DAP) during 2007/2008 season. There were no significant differences in soil water extraction by cropping systems in the whole profile during both cropping seasons. Intercropping of sunflower resulted in grain yield reduction of sunflower of up to 50 and 30% of cowpea during 2007/2008 and 2008/2009, respectively. Water use and water use efficiency by SS were significantly greater than other cropping systems during the second cropping season.

Keywords: Cowpea, Intercropping, Semi-arid, Sunflower, Water use

1. Introduction

Sunflower (*Helianthus annuus* L.) is the most important oilseed crop in South Africa. It is the third largest grain crop produced in South Africa after maize (*Zea mays*) and wheat (*Triticum aestivum*) [1]. Sunflower seed is utilized in the manufacture of sunflower oil and oilcake for animal feed. Sunflower is adapted in both hot and dry climate. This makes Limpopo Province ideal for growing the sunflower crop [2]. However, its production in the semi-arid area is limited by variable and low rainfall amount. Soil moisture loss is further exacerbated by evaporation due to high temperatures during the growing season [3]. Soil moisture loss under these conditions is further worsened by the fact that sunflower residue is fragile and does not provide adequate ground cover [4]. However, research has shown that legumes such as cowpea (*Vigna unguiculata*) intercropped in sunflower could increase soil cover and suppress soil moisture loss by evaporation [5]. Furthermore, previous research has shown that intercrops can improve water use efficiency [6, 7].

Cowpea is an important food and fodder legume crop in the semi-arid tropics, South Africa included. Being a drought tolerant and warm weather crop, cowpea is well adapted to the drier regions of the tropics where other food legumes do not perform well. It can fix atmospheric nitrogen through its nodules. It is reported that about 30 kg N ha^{-1} can be contributed to the soil by cowpea. The amount of N fixed is a function of cowpea cultivar [4]. It grows well in poor soils with high sand content, little organic matter, and low phosphorus content, such as those found in smallholder farming sector of the Limpopo Province. Also, it is shade tolerant and therefore, compatible as an intercrop with several field crops, including sunflower. Its rapid growth habit and quick ground cover prevents soil erosion. Furthermore, the in-situ decay of its roots and nitrogen-rich residues improves soil fertility and soil structure. These qualities have made cowpea an important component of the subsistence agriculture particularly in the dry savannas of the sub-Saharan Africa [8]. Cowpea is important to food security in less developed countries of the tropics particularly Asia and Africa. As a vegetable, it is consumed as young leaves, green pods, and green seeds. In addition, dry seeds are used in various food preparations. Its high protein content (>25%) in its seeds and tender leaves makes it ideal diet for the rural and urban poor whose diet consists of starchy foods [5]. Apart from improving the diet of the rural poor, it is envisaged that the sunflower and cowpea crop mixtures could also offer advantages, such as, yield advantage [9, 10], yield stability [11], and better weed control [12].

Cowpea and groundnut (*Arachis hypogeae*) are often grown as intercrops among smallholder farmers of the Limpopo Province. However, little scientific research has been conducted to quantify the agronomic value of this practice [13]. Sunflower is grown mainly as a sole crop under commercial production [14]. Its cultivation by the smallholder farming sector is little known. However, sunflower crop has a potential in smallholder farming sector if integrated into the existing traditional farming systems which are based on growing crops in mixtures [8]. There is evidence of sunflower production in mixtures by the smallholder farmers in the Limpopo Province. However, no scientific research is documented. In particular, there is no information on the productivity of sunflower × cowpea intercropping systems. There is a need therefore to evaluate the productivity of sunflower and cowpea mixtures in order to optimize their production. The major objectives of this chapter are to compare (i) the changes in soil profile water storage, (ii) water use efficiency, and (ii) productivity of the three cropping systems under semi-arid conditions of South Africa.

2. Trial site

A 2-year field experiment was conducted during 2007/2008 and 200820/09 growing seasons at the University of Venda in Thohoyandou, South Africa (22°58′S, 30°26′E). Altitude is 596 m above sea level. The terrain is characterized by a slope of 8%. The daily temperatures at Thohoyandou vary from about 25 to 40°C in summer and between approximately 12 and 26°C in winter. Rainfall is highly seasonal occurs between October and March. Crop failure and low yields are associated with midsummer drought [15]. Rainfall varies temporarily and ranges between 500 and 800 mm per year. The study site is characterized by deep and red clayey classified as Rhodic Ferralsols [16]. The soil is composed of 10% sand, 30% silt, and 60% clay. Soil pH is low (pH 5.5). Selected chemical and physical soil properties were previously presented in [17].

2.1 Trial description

The experiment was conducted during 2007/2008 and 200820/09 growing seasons. The trial was complete randomized block design (CRBD) with four replications under conventional tillage (CT). The field was disk ploughed and disk harrowed at the start of the trial. The plots were hand dug to a depth of 20 cm the following season. Three cropping systems consisting of sole sunflower (SS), sole cowpea (SC), and sunflower–cowpea intercrop (ISC) were laid out in 9 m × 10 m plots. Sunflower hybrid (cv. AFG 5551) and local cowpea landrace were planted. The intercrop components were sown manually using row replacement series (1:1) using tramline row spacing (1 m × 2 m). Final sunflower plant population was 30,000 plants ha^{-1} while that for cowpea was 66,666 plants ha^{-1}. This gave the intercrop density of 48,333 plants ha^{-1}. A commercial fertilizer was incorporated a rate of 33 kg N ha^{-1}, 50 kg P ha^{-1}, and 33 kg K ha^{-1}. In the second season, the same fertilizer rate was repeated with an additional 178 kg ha $^{-1}$ limestone ammonium nitrate (LAN) (28) as top dressing on sunflower 5 weeks after planting. Weeding was done manually using hand hoes during the season. Plots were kept clean during fallow period by using glysphosphate (360 g/l). Malathion 50% EC (a.i. Merkaptotion 500 g/l; Mercaptothion 500 g/l) was used to control aphids and beetles.

2.2. Data collection and analysis

2.2.1. Grain yield

Sunflower was harvested at physiological maturity at 87 and 79 days after planting (DAP) during 2007/2008 and 2008/2009 seasons, respectively, by cutting 6-m length of the central rows. The heads were air-dried in the shed. Cowpeas were harvested at 150 and 140 DAP during 2007/2008 and 2008/2009 seasons, respectively, from 4 m^2 (2 m × 2 m). The air- dried cowpea grain was separated from the stalks weighed and oven-dried at 70°C for 24 h. The grain yield was adapted to 13% moisture content.

2.2.2. *Soil profile soil storage*

Volumetric water content of the soil profile was determined on weekly basis using a calibrated neutron water meter (NWM) (Campbell Pacific Nuclear International 503DR). Galvanized access tubes measuring 50 mm in diameter were inserted to a depth of 1500 mm. Two access tubes were inserted per plot between the 1-m crop rows. Readings were taken in depth increments of 300 mm until 1500 mm. Standard counts (C_s) of the NWM were determined in five replicates. Soil water content was calculated using the following calibration equations developed on site:

$$\theta_{v0-300} = 0.4339 \times CR - 0.2893 \left(R^2 = 0.998 \right) \quad (1)$$

$$\theta_{v300-900} = 0.2678 \times CR - 0.0378 \left(R^2 = 0.921 \right) \quad (2)$$

$$\theta_{v900-1500} = 0.6331 \times CR - 0.5077 \ (R^2 = 0.956) \quad (3)$$

where θ_{v0-300} is the volumetric water content in the soil layer 0–300 mm (mm^{-1} mm^{-1}), CR is the count ratio calculated as count/standard count (C_s). Soil water storage (mm) was calculated by multiplying volumetric water content by soil layer thickness (mm).

2.2.3. *Water use and water use efficiency*

Water balance was calculated by the following equation:

$$P = R + D + ET + \Delta W \quad (4)$$

where P is precipitation (mm); R is surface runoff (mm); D is deep drainage (mm); ET is evapotranspiration or water use (mm); and ΔW is change of soil water content (mm). The sum of runoff (R) and deep drainage (D) were assumed to be zero during the experimental period, simplifying Eq. (4) as follows:

$$ET = -\Delta W + P \quad (5)$$

Precipitation was measured using an automatic weather station which was located 20 m away from the experimental block. Water use efficiency was calculated using the water balance equation, assuming no drainage, and runoff water, as follows:

$$WUE = Y / ET \quad (6)$$

where WUE is the water use efficiency (kg ha^{-1} mm^{-1}); Y is the grain yield (kg ha^{-1}); and ET is the total evapotranspiration over the growing season (mm). Similarly, intercrop WUE was calculated on the basis of total grain yield of sunflower and cowpea.

2.2.4. Land equivalent ratio

Land equivalent ratio (LER) was calculated according to [18] as follows:

$$LER_T = LER_S + LER_C \tag{7}$$

where LER_T = total land equivalent ratio and, LER_S = partial LER for sunflower per unit area; LER_C = partial LER for cowpeas per unit area.

Partial LER is defined as the ratio of yield per unit area of the specific intercrop (Yi) versus the mono-crop (Y_m) that is as follows:

$$\text{Partial LER} = Yi / Y_m \tag{8}$$

If $LER_T > 1$, intercropping has a yield advantage, if $LER_T < 1$, there is yield disadvantage from intercropping, and when $LER_T = 1$, there is no advantage to intercropping [10].

3. Results

3.1. Variation of soil profile water storage

Rainfall amounting to 391 mm was recorded over 2007/2008 experimental period. Most of the rainfall was >10 mm and accounted for 93% (365 mm) of the total rainfall while the rest were <10 mm. Most of the rainfall, this season occurred in January and was followed by dry spells in February and March. Due to the breakdown of the NWM water measurements started 21 DAP. Soil water content variations in 0–300, 300–600, 600–900, 900–1200, and 1200–1500 mm layers measured in 2007/2008 season for the three cropping systems are shown in **Figure 1**. Soil water content was high at 21 DAP and started to decline until 63 DAP for all cropping systems. The profile water storage decreased in all cropping systems. During this vegetative period, the soil profile received rainfall events below 10 mm. There were no significant differences among cropping systems in the 0–300 mm layer. This top layer was characterized by variations in water content, possibly as a result of evaporation and root uptake. Similarly, the layers 300–600 and 600–900 mm showed no significant differences in water extraction patterns during this period. However, significant differences in soil water content were observed at 35 DAP in the 900–1200 mm layer. There intercrop recorded more water extraction than the SS and SC. There were significant differences in water uptake at DAP 56, 63, and 70 in the 1200–1500 mm layer. The SS used more water than the SC and the intercrop.

The SC had the least water consumption. The highest rainfall amount of 70 mm was received at flowering stage (after DAP 70). This resulted in the increase in soil profile water content. The increase was more pronounced in the 0–300 and 300–600 mm layers. There were more fluctuations of soil water content in the 0–300 and 300–600 mm layer compared to other layers. However, the 0–300 mm layer had marked fluctuations. There were no significant differences in water consumption in the 0–300 and 300–600 mm layers until DAS 119. At DAP 112 (grain filling stage) the intercrop extracted more water compared to other cropping systems in the 600–900 mm layer. Between DAP 56 and 119, the SS crop significantly extracted more water compared to the other cropping systems in the 1200–1500 mm layers. Total soil water extraction by SC was less compared to the other cropping systems but the differences were not statistically significant ($P < 0.05$) (**Figure 2**).

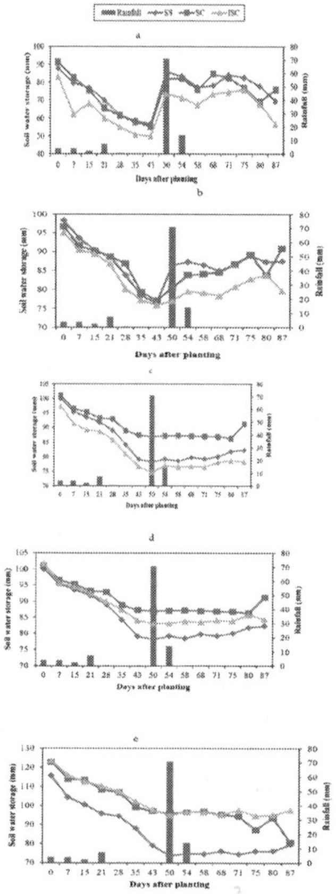

Figure 1. Soil water storage in various layers (a = 0–300; b = 300–600; c = 600–900; d = 900–1200; e = 1200–1500 mm) during the 2007/2008 for sole sunflower (SS), sole cowpea (SC), and sunflower × cowpea intercrop (ISC).

http://dx.doi.org/10.5772/62764

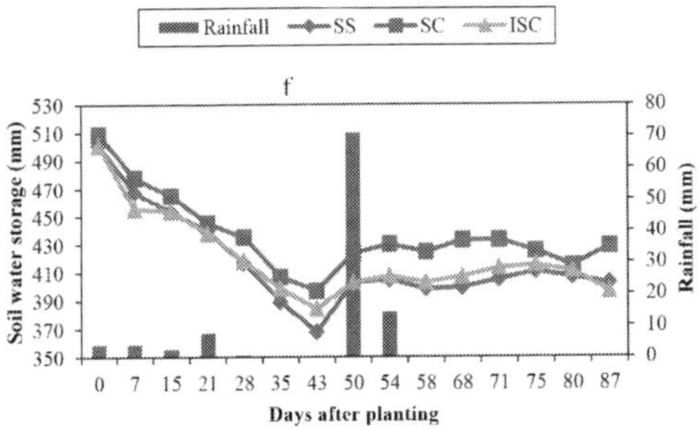

Figure 2. Soil water storage in total soil profile (f = 0–1500 mm) during the 2007/2008 for sole sunflower (SS), sole cowpea (SC) and sunflower × cowpea intercrop (ISC).

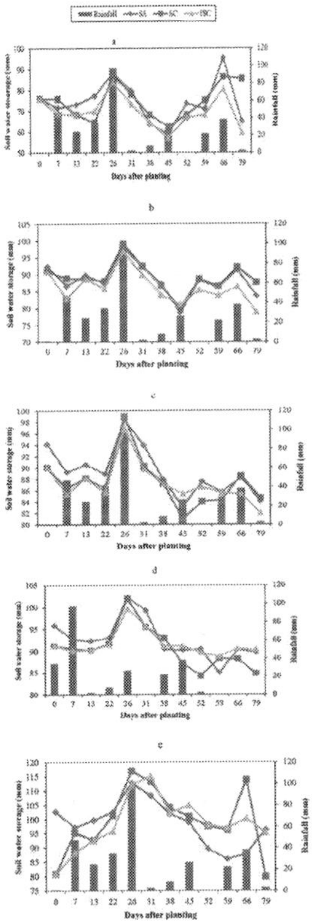

Figure 3. Soil water storage in various layers (a = 0–300; b = 300–600; c = 600–900; d = 900–1200; e = 1200–1500 mm) during the 2008/2009 for sole sunflower (SS), sole cowpea (SC), and sunflower × cowpea intercrop (ISC).

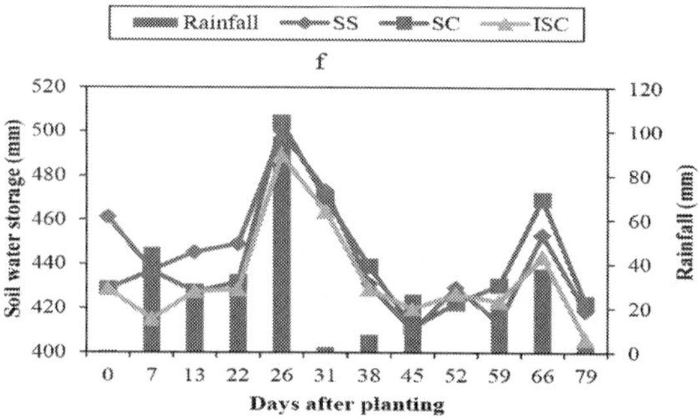

Figure 4. Soil water storage in total soil profile (f = 0–1500 mm) during the 2008/2009 for sole sunflower (SS), sole cowpea (SC), and sunflower × cowpea intercrop (ISC).

Compared to the 2007/2008, the rainfall during 2008/2009 (405 mm) was well distributed. **Figure 3** shows soil water content in various layers for the 2008/2009 growing season. The 0–300 mm layer showed huge variations in soil water content which increased soon after rainfall. The SS extracted significantly less soil water from the 0 to 300 mm layer compared to the other cropping systems at DAP 22. Thereafter, there was no systematic water extraction pattern recorded in the period DAP 66–79. By the end of this period the intercrop had the highest extraction followed by SC and the lowest SS ($P < 0.001$). Cropping system water extraction pattern in the 0–300 mm layer was similar to 300–600, 600–900, and 900–1200 mm layers. There was no clear water extraction pattern in the 1200–1500 mm layer by all cropping systems. Similarly, no systematic soil water extraction was observed in the whole profile from the beginning to the end of the 2008/2009 growing season (**Figure 4**).

3.2. Productivity of cropping systems

The yield of sole and intercrop sunflower increased during season 2008/2009 compared to 2007/2008 while the yield of SC and its intercrop decreased in the same period (**Table 1**). The yield of each crop species was not significantly different during 2007/2008 season. However, a statistical difference of yield was observed in both crop species during 2008/2009.

The intercrop was more productive than the sole crops ($LER_T > 1$) (**Table 2**). The highest sunflower yield loss of nearly 50% was recorded during 2007/2008 season, while 31% yield loss in cowpea was recorded during 2008/2009 season. The cowpea was a better competitor for resources in 2007/2008 season ($LER_C = 0.86$) but the sunflower exhibited higher competitive ability than cowpea during 2008/2009 season ($LER_S = 0.80$).

3.3. Water use and water use efficiency

Water use by all cropping systems was higher during 2008/2009 compared to 2007/2008 (**Table 3**). There was no statistical difference in water consumption between the cropping systems during 2007/2008 season. However, water consumption by SS was statistical greater than SC and the intercrop during 2008/2009 season. Water use efficiency by the SS and intercrop increased during 2007/2008 compared to 2008/2009. The WUE by the cowpea decreased by nearly 50% during 2008/2009 compared to 2007/2008. WUE by SS was significantly higher compared to the other cropping systems during 2007/2008 season. During 2008/2009, WUE by all cropping systems was significantly different from each other. The SS had the highest WUE then the intercrop and SC in that order (**Table 4**).

Cropping system	**Yield (kg ha^{-1})**	
	2007/2008	**2008/2009**
Sole sunflower	1135	1203
Sole cowpea	256	137
Intercrop sunflower	584	960
Intercrop cowpea	221	95

Table 1. Mean grain yield for different cropping systems during the 2007/2008 and 2008/2009 seasons.

LER	**Growing season**	
	2007/2008	**2008/2009**
LER_S	0.51	0.80
LER_C	0.86	0.69
LER_T	1.37	1.49

Table 2. LER during 2007/2008 and 2008/2009 seasons.

Cropping system	**Water use (mm)**	
	2007/2008	**2008/2009**
Sole sunflower	475.5	455.4
Sole cowpea	401.8	406.6
Intercrop	415.5	433.7

Table 3. Water use (WU) of crops in different cropping systems during the 2007/2008 and 2008/2009 seasons.

Cropping system	**WUE (kg ha^{-1} mm^{-1})**	
	2007/2008	**2008/2009**
Sole sunflower	2.40	3.53
Sole cowpea	0.62	0.34
Intercrop	1.94	2.51

Table 4. Water use efficiency (WUE) of crops in different cropping systems during the 2007/2008 and 2008/2009 seasons.

4. Discussion

Low rainfall during 2007/2008 season resulted in continuous decline of soil profile water content until DAP 63. This happened during the vegetative period when the crops needed water for development. High amount of rainfall received during 2008/2008 season could be attributed to better performance especially of sunflower crop species during this season compared to the previous one. However, there were no significant differences in total profile water extraction all by all cropping systems during the two seasons.

Water extraction patterns were almost similar for all cropping systems in the 0–300 and 300–600 mm layers during season 2007/2008. The intercrop extracted slightly higher soil water than other cropping systems throughout the rest of the season. An almost similar trend was observed during 2008/2009 season in all cropping systems in the same soil layers. However, extraction patterns by all cropping systems in the 0–300 and 300–600 mm layers were statistically non- significant. The intercrop did not extract greater moisture as expected. Similar findings were reported in maize-bean intercrop [19]. Similar moisture extraction was observed in the 600–900 mm layer (**Figure 1**). However, water extraction by the intercrop was significant at 112 DAP during 2007/2008.

In the lower profile soil layers (900–1200 and 1200–1500 mm for 2007/2008), the sunflower extracted significantly more soil water compared to other cropping systems after 56 and 66 DAP during 2007/2008 and 2008/2009, respectively. This was not unexpected. The sunflower crop has a deeper and extensive rooting system that is able to exploit water from deeper soil layers [20]. Despite the differences in tillage systems, our results are analogous to those of [20] who demonstrated that the average soil profile water content at harvest under sunflower was lower (77 mm) than that under cowpea (158 mm) in no-till (NT) and stubble mulch tillage in a clay loam soil.

Good rainfall conditions were attributed to the higher sole and intercrop sunflower yield during 2008/2009 compared to 2007/2008 (**Table 1**). Significant difference in yield between the sole and intercrop sunflower was observed during 2008/2009 season. Similar results were reported in other cropping systems. Higher sunflower yield in sole crop compared to its mixture with soybean were reported [21]. Differences in yield in the sole and intercropped sunflower were attributed to competition for resources such as nutrients and moisture. Higher productivity of SS over its intercrop in the current study was attributed to lower population in the intercrop. The results could also suggest intense competition between crop species in the crop mixture. It was reported that some cowpea genotypes can suppress the growth of sunflower [22]. In contrast, the grain yield of cowpea showed no statistical difference due to cropping system probably because cowpea was able to out-compete sunflower in acquiring nutrients and other resources. However, cowpea was a better competitor than sunflower during 2007/2008 season as indicated by the LER_C (**Table 2**). Overall, the values of LER during the two seasons were >1, indicating that the intercrop was more productive than the pure stands of sunflower and cowpea as earlier reported in other intercrops [18].

The observed greater WU in SS compared to the cowpea and intercrops was attributed to the relatively higher WU of sunflower compared to the cowpea as previously reported [23]. When the two crops were combined in an intercrop their combined WU became higher than the SC. Similar findings have been reported [23]. The SS exhibited greater WUE than other cropping systems. The intercrop was second followed by the SC. Conflicting results on WU and WUE of crop mixtures have been reported by other researchers. It was reported that WUE of maize-bean intercropping were equal or higher than maize sole crops, and higher than bean sole cropping [24]. In Nigeria, [25] reported that intercropping cowpea with millet did not increase WUE over the sole millet. Results in the current study indicated that under high rainfall conditions WUE by cowpea was significantly reduced. This could mean that the cowpea crop was better able to utilize limited soil moisture, thus making it an ideal crop in water scarce environments such as those prevailing at the study site.

5. Conclusion

Soil water extraction patterns could be related to seasonal rainfall conditions and cropping systems. Soil moisture extraction patterns by layers showed no significant differences in all cropping systems in the 0–300, 300–600, and 600–900 mm during 2007/2008 and 2008/2009 seasons. SS significantly extracted more soil water than SC and the intercrop from the 1200 to 1500 mm layer after 56 DAP during 2007/2008 season. Overall, the whole profile did not show statistical difference in moisture depletion by crops and their combinations during the two seasons. Intercropping of sunflower resulted in grain yield reduction of sunflower of 50% and 30% of cowpea during 2007/2008 and 2008/2009, respectively. LER > 1 meant that intercropping was advantageous in the utilization of environmental resources. Generally, WU and WUE by SS were significantly greater than other cropping systems during the second cropping season (2008/2009). The SC had the lowest WU and WUE.

Acknowledgements

This study was supported by International Foundation for Science (Sweden) Grant No. C/3918-1. We appreciate the field assistance offered by Mrs. Memory Mzezewa.

Author details

Jestinos Mzezewa[1*] and Eastonce T. Gwata[2]

*Address all correspondence to: Jestinos.Mzezewa@univen.ac.za

1 Department of Soil Science, University of Venda, P/Bag X5050, Thohoyandou, South Africa

2 Department of Plant Production, University of Venda, P/Bag X5050, Thohoyandou, South Africa

References

[1] Sunflower seed. Grains South Africa 2003 [Internet]. Available from: http://www.grainsa.co.za [Accessed: 2015-12-10].

[2] Thomas R. Crop Production in the Limpopo Province. In: Nesamvuni AE, Oni SA, Odhiambo JJO, Nthakheni ND, editors. Agriculture as the cornerstone of the economy in the Limpopo Province. A study commissioned by the Economic Cluster of the Limpopo Provincial Government under the leadership of the Department of Agriculture. Department of Agriculture, Limpopo Province, 2013. p. 50–65.

[3] Bennie ATP, Hensley M. Maximizing precipitation utilization in dryland agriculture in South Africa—a review. Journal of Hydrology. 2001;241:124–139.

[4] Kendel HJ, Schneiter AA, Johnson BL. Intercropping legumes into sunflower at different growth stages. Crop Science. 1997;37:1532–1537.

[5] Walker S, Ogindo HO. The water budget of rainfed maize and bean intercrop. Physics and Chemistry of the Earth, Parts A/B/C. 2003;28:(20–27):919–926.

[6] Reddy MS, Willey RW. Growth and resource-use studies in an intercrop of pearl millet/groundnut. Field Crops Research. 1981;4:13–24.

[7] Morris RA, Garrity DP. Resource capture and utilization in intercropping: Water. Field Crops Research. 1993;34:303–317.

[8] Ofori F, Stern WR. Cereal–legume intercropping systems. Advances in Agronomy. 1987;41:41–90.

[9] Willey RW. Intercropping-its importance and research needs. Part 1. Competition and yield advantages. Field Crops Abstracts. 1979;32:1–10.

[10] Willey RW. Resource use in intercropping systems. Agricultural Water Management. 1990;17:215–231.

[11] Filho JMPL. Physiological responses of maize and cowpea to intercropping. Pesquisa Agropecuaria Brasileira. 2000;35(5):1–15.

[12] Aladesanwa RD, Adigun AW. Evaluation of sweet potato (*Ipomea batatas*) live mulch at different spacings for weed suppression and yield response of maize (*Zea mays* L.) in southwestern Nigeria. Crop Protection. 2008;27:968–975.

[13] Ayisi KK, Mpangane PNZ, Whitbread A. Grain yield and symbiotic activity of cowpea cultivars grown in sole and intercropping systems with maize in the Limpopo Province o South Africa [Internet]. 2004. Available from: http://www.cropscience.org.au/icsc2004/poster/2/1/2/133_ayisikkv.htm [Accessed: 2015-11-20].

[14] Botha JJ. Evaluation of Maize and sunflower production in semi-arid area using in-field rainwater harvesting [thesis]. Bloemfontein: University of the Free State, South Africa, 2006.

[15] Beukes DJ, Bennie ATP, Hensley M. Optimization of soil water use in the dry crop production areas of South Africa. In: Proceedings of the 1998 workshops of the Optimizing Soil Water Use (OSWU) consortium: Efficient soil water use: The key to sustainable crop production in dry areas of West Asia, and North and sub-Saharan Africa (Niger) (April 26–30) and 1999 (Jordan) (May 9–13). Aleppo, Syria: ICARDA; Patancheru, India: ICRISAT. p. 165–191.

[16] World Reference Base for Soil Resources. A Framework for International Classification, Correlation and Communication, Rome, 2006. World Soil Resources Rep.103. IUSS/ISRIC/FAO.

[17] Mzezewa J, Misi T, Van Rensburg LD. Characterisation of rainfall at a semi-arid ecotope in the Limpopo Province (South Africa) and its implications for sustainable crop production. Water SA. 2010;36(1):19–26.

[18] Mead R, Willey RW. The concept of 'Land Equivalent Ratio' and advantages in yields from intercropping. Experimental Agriculture. 1980;16:217–228.

[19] Ogindo HO, Walker S. Comparison of measured changes in seasonal soil water content by rainfed maize-bean intercrop and component cropping systems in a semi-arid region of southern Africa. Physics and Chemistry of the Earth. 2005;30:799–808.

[20] Moroke TS, Schwartz RC, Brown, KW, Juo ASR. Water use efficiency of dryland cowpea, sorghum and sunflower under reduced tillage. Soil and Tillage Research. 2005;112:76–84.

[21] Khan A, Khan S, Asrar M, Khan M. Efficiency of intercropping maize, soyabean and sunflower on grain yield. Pakistan Journal of Biological Sciences. 1999;2(4):1611–1613.

[22] Wang G, Ehlers JD, Ogbuchiekwe EJ, Yang S, Mcgiffen ME. Competitiveness of erect, semierect, and prostrate cowpea genotypes with sunflower (*Hellianthus annuus*) and purslane (*Portulaca oleracea*). Weed Science. 2004;52:815–820.

[23] Moroke TS, Schwartz RC, Brown KW, Juo ASR. Soil water depletion and root distribution of three dryland crops. Soil Sci Soc. Am. J. 2005;69:197–205.

[24] Tsubo M, Mukhala E, Ogindo HO, Walker S. Productivity of sunflower-bean intercropping in a semi-arid region of South Africa. Water SA. 2003;29(4):381–388.

[25] Grema AK, Hess TM. Water balance and water use of pearl millet-cowpea intercrops in north east Nigeria. Agricultural Water Management. 1994;26(3):169–185.

Chapter 8

Herbicide and Cover Crop Residue Integration in Conservation Tillage Tomato

Andrew J. Price, Jessica Kelton and Lina Sarunaite

Additional information is available at the end of the chapter

http://dx.doi.org/10.5772/62320

Abstract

The increased adoption of conservation tillage in vegetable production requires more information on the role of various cover crops in weed control, tomato quality, and yield. Three conservation-tillage systems utilizing crimson clover, turnip, and cereal rye as winter cover crops were compared to a conventional black polythene mulch system, with or without herbicide, for weed control and tomato yield. All cover crops were flattened with a mechanical roller/crimper prior to chemical desiccation. Herbicide treatments included a PRE application of S-metolachlor (1.87 kg a.i. ha^{-1}) either alone, or followed by an early POST metribuzin (0.56 kg a.i. ha^{-1}) application followed by a late POST application of clethodim (0.28 kg a.i. ha^{-1}). Except for spotted spurge and tall morningglory only the main effect of herbicide treatments and cover crops affected weed control. For the majority of the weeds, no significant differences in weed control were observed with rye residue and plastic mulch treatments; however, turnip and crimson clover residue failed to control most weeds. Rye residue provided 86% large crabgrass, 80% goosegrass and 84% Broadleaf signalgrass control. Yellow nutsedge was controlled 65% by plastic mulch and only 60% by Rye residue. Pokeweed was controlled 80% by plastic mulch treatment. *S*-metolachlor applied PRE was sufficient in controlling leafy spurge and tall morningglory in plastic mulch and rye residue plots. Yield was less following either crimson clover or turnip cover crops compared to rye or the polythene mulch system. Application of herbicides resulted in better yields compared to the no-herbicide treatments. Economic analysis indicated that there was no significant difference between using a rye cover crop or plastic under any of the alternative herbicide treatment regimes in 2005. This research demonstrates the possibility of growing tomato in conservation tillage systems using high residue cover crops and herbicides to maintain season long weed control.

Keywords: conservation agriculture, cover crop, fruit, conservation tillage, weed suppression, vegetable

Nomenclature

S-metolachlor; metribuzin; clethodim; broadleaf signalgrass, *Brachiaria* platyphylla, BRAPP; large crabgrass, *Digitaria sanguinalis* DIGSA; leafy spurge, *Euphorbia esula* L. EPHES; common pokeweed, *Phytolaca americana*, PHATAM; yellow nutsedge, *Cyperus esculentus* L.CYPES; tomato, *Lycopersicon esculentum* L.; crimson clover, *Trifolium incarnatum* L.; rye, *Secale cereale* L.; turnip, *Brassica rapa* L.

Abbreviations

PRE, preemergence;

POST, postemergence

Tomato (*Lycopersicon esculentum* L.) is the most popular fruit in the world. Nearly 1.7 million tons of fresh market field grown tomatoes were produced in the U.S. in 2005 [1]. The U.S. produces more than 11% of the world's tomato crop. Tomato production systems typically utilize conventional tillage, a bedded plastic mulch culture, and multiple herbicide applications to control weeds. These conventional tillage systems enhance soil erosion and nutrient loss by reducing rainfall infiltration [2]. Additionally, tillage increases aeration which increases the rate of organic matter mineralization in the surface soil, thus reducing soil organic matter content, soil cation exchange capacity, and potential productivity [3, 4].

Plastic mulch can increase soil temperature which can expedite tomato harvest earliness [5]. Tomato harvest was not early following a hairy vetch mulch system [6, 7]. The use of plastic mulches in sustainable or organic production systems is in question by some producers and consumers since the mulch itself is non-biodegradable and made of non-renewable resources. Another environmental disadvantage with using plastic mulch vs. organic mulches is increased chemical runoff from plastic mulch systems and subsequent offsite chemical loading [8]. Thus, the intensive use of pesticides in vegetable production has resulted in ecological concerns. Therefore, alternative production practices that reduce tomato production inputs while maintaining yield and quality are desired.

One alternative for alleviating the aforementioned concerns is the use of high residue cover crops combined with reduced tillage. Cover crops in conservation-tillage systems can be terminated during early reproductive growth by mechanically rolling and treating with burndown herbicides to leave a dense mat of residue (>4,500 kg ha^{-1}) on the soil surface into which cash crops are planted [9, 10]. Adoption of high residue cover crops is increasing in southeastern US corn (*Zea mays* L.) and cotton (*Gossypium hirsutum* L.) row crop systems [11–13]. Because the southeastern US typically receives adequate rainfall in the winter months, timely planted winter cover crops can attain relatively high maturity and biomass before termination. Cover crops can enhance the overall productivity and soil quality by increasing organic matter and nitrogen content [14], as well as aid in water conservation by increasing soil water infiltration rates [15]. Additionally, previous research has also focused on weed control provided by high residue cover crops in both field and vegetable crops [11, 16, 17].

Winter cover crop biomass can affect subsequent early season weed control [18–20]. Cover crop residue facilitates weed control by providing an unfavorable environment for weed germination and establishment under the residue, as well as allelopathy [21, 22]. Teasdale and Daughtry [23] reported 52–70% reduction in weed biomass with live hairy vetch cover crop compared to a fallow treatment owing to changes in light and soil temperature regimen under the vetch canopy. Teasdale and Mohler [21] reported that legume mulches such as crimson clover and hairy vetch (*Vicia villosa* Roth) suppressed redroot pigweed (*Amaranthus retrofloxus* L.) at an exponential rate as a function of residue biomass.

However, adoption of cover crops in tomato production has been limited because (1) currently available transplanters have problems penetrating heavy residue and (2) heavy cover crop residue can intercept delivery of soil-active herbicides. Research in the last two decades has extensively debated the advantages and disadvantages of cover crops vs. conventional plastic mulch systems for tomato production. Better or comparable tomato yields with hairy vetch cover crop system have been reported compared to the conventional polyethylene mulch system [24, 25]. Akemo et al. [26] also reported higher tomato yield with spring sown cover crops than the conventionally cultivated check. Weed control with cover crops however varies with cover crop species, amount of residue produced, and environmental conditions. Teasdale [21] reported that biomass levels achieved by cover crops before termination was sufficient only for early season weed control. Supplemental weed control measures are usually required to achieve season long weed control and to avoid yield losses [16, 27].

Cereal rye and crimson clover are two common winter cover crops widely used in the southeastern U.S. Both cover crops contain allelopathic compounds and produce residues that inhibit weed growth [28, 29]. Brassica cover crops are relatively new in the southeastern US but, are becoming increasingly popular due to their potential allelopathic effects. Therefore, the objectives of this research were to evaluate: 1) weed control in three different high residue cover crop conservation tillage systems utilizing the Brazilian cover crop management system, and 2) tomato stand establishment, yield, and net returns of conservation-transplanted tomatoes compared to the polythene mulch system following three different herbicide management systems.

1. Materials and methods

1.1. Field experiment

The experiment was established in autumn 2004 and 2005 at the North Alabama Horticulture Experiment Station, Cullman, AL on a Hartsell fine sandy loam soil (Fine-loamy, siliceous, sub-active, thermic Typic Hapludults). The experimental design was a randomized complete block with four replicates. Plot size at both locations was 1.8 by 6 m containing a single row of tomatoes with a 0.5 m spacing between plants.

The three winter cover crops [cereal rye cv Elbon, crimson clover cv AU Robin and turnip (*Brassica rapa* L subsp. *rapa* cv Civastro)] were compared to black polythene mulch for their weed suppressive potential and effect on yield and grade of fresh market tomatoes. Winter cover crops were planted with a no till drill each fall. Rye was seeded at a rate of 100 kg ha^{-1}, whereas clover and turnip were seeded at 28 kg ha^{-1}. Nitrogen was applied at a rate of 67 kg ha^{-1} on rye and turnip plots in early spring of each year. Cover crops were terminated at flowering stage in late spring. To determine winter cover crop biomass production, plants were clipped at ground level from one randomly selected 0.25 m^2 area per replicate immediately before termination. Plant samples were dried at 65°C for 72 hours and weighed. Cover crops were terminated with a mechanical roller crimper prior to an application of glyphosate at 1.12 kg a.e. ha^{-1}. The rolling process produced a uniform residue cover over the plots.

All four cover systems (three winter cover crops plus plastic mulch) were evaluated with and without herbicide for weed control. Herbicide treatments included a preemergence (PRE) application of *S*-metolachlor (1.87 kg a.i. ha^{-1}) either alone or followed by an early postemergence (EPOST) metribuzin (0.56 kg a.i. ha^{-1}) application, followed by a late POST (LPOST) application of clethodim (0.28 kg a.i. ha^{-1}). These three herbicide treatments were applied in a factorial combination with the four mulch treatments. Additionally, a fallow no herbicide treatment plot was included in each replication. The PRE application occurred one day before transplanting, the EPOST application was applied two weeks after transplanting, and the LPOST application was delayed until tomatoes were near mid-bloom. The PRE herbicide treatment in plastic mulch plots were applied before laying the plastic on top of the beds and POST treatments were applied over the total surface of the beds including tomato plant openings. Tomato cv. 'Florida 47' seedlings were transplanted on 4th April 2005 and on April 9th in 2006.

Tomato seedlings were planted with a modified RJ No-till transplanter (RJ Equipment, Blenhiem, Ontario, Canada), which included a subsoiler shank installed to penetrate the heavy residue and disrupt a naturally occurring compacted soil layer found at both experimental sites at a depth of 30–40 cm. Additionally, two driving wheels were utilized (one wheel on each side of the tomato row) instead of the original single wheel at the center of the row, to improve stability and eliminate drive wheel re-compaction of the soil opening created by the shank. The plastic-mulch plots were conventionally tilled utilizing a tractor mounted rototiller prior to bedding and plastic installation; tomatoes were hand transplanted in the plastic mulch each year. Water was applied to all the plots immediately after transplanting. Thereafter, plots were irrigated every other day using a surface drip tape. General production practices included staking and fertilization. Fertilizer 13-13-13 was applied prior to planting achieving 448 kg of N ha^{-1} and then 7.8 kg of calcium nitrate ha^{-1} was applied once every week with the irrigation system.

Weed control was evaluated by visual ratings (0% = no control, 100% = complete control) 28 days after treatment (DAT) of the EPOST herbicide application. All weed species present were evaluated for control (as a reduction in total above ground biomass resulting from both reduced emergence and growth). Stand establishment was determined by counting the number of living tomato plants in each plot two weeks after LPOST application. Ripe tomatoes were hand harvested from the entire plot area in weekly intervals and sorted according to size (small, medium, large, and extra large categories).

http://dx.doi.org/10.5772/62320

1.2. Statistical analysis

Non-normality and heterogeneous variances were encountered with percent control data. Various approaches were tried to alleviate these statistical problems and the arcsine transformation was deemed the best compromise between achieving normality of residuals and among treatment homogeneity of variances. The transformed data were subjected to mixed models analysis of variance as implemented in JMP statistical software. Years, herbicide treatments and ground cover treatments were considered fixed effects while their interaction with treatment replication was considered random effects. Differences between treatments means were determined by Fisher's protected LSD ($\alpha = 0.05$) where year by treatment interactions were not significant data pooled across years.

1.3. Economic analysis

Enterprise budgets were generated using Mississippi State (2005) vegetable planning budgets [30]. These budgets were based on a standard yield of 39,230 kg ha^{-1} (35,000 lbs ac^{-1}). Seed and plant costs include the cost of cover crop seed (Turnip—$146 ha^{-1}; Crimson Clover—$58 ha^{-1}; Rye—$49 ha^{-1}) and the cost of tomato transplants ($838 ha^{-1}). Fertilizer costs included the cost of N application and calcium nitrate for the cash crop ($228 ha^{-1}), as well as, the additional N applied for the rye and turnip cover crops ($68 ha^{-1}). Herbicide costs were based on treatment applications as described above and varies with cover crop x herbicide treatment combinations. Insecticide and fungicide costs followed extension recommendations and varied by year due to different climatic conditions (i.e. insecticide and fungicide costs were $122 ha^{-1} and $189 ha^{-1} in 2006, respectively). Harvesting costs are based on custom rates for harvesting, packing, and grading of tomatoes based on hand harvesting. Supplies costs represent purchase of stakes, string, buckets, as well as other harvesting and planting supplies. Irrigation costs are broken into the variable cost of water application ($26 ha^{-1}) and the fixed costs of the machinery ($1890 ha^{-1}). Irrigation costs were calculated based on the cost of surface drip tape and pumping 152 mm of water every week from surface water reservoirs located on both experiment stations.

Machinery costs are broken into variable and fixed costs. Variable machinery costs represent the cost fuel, as well as repair and maintenance costs. Fixed machinery costs represent cost of machinery purchase based on an annual payment of loan, interest, taxes, and depreciation. Labor costs represent operator labor for machinery, as well as hand labor in the field. Equipment used during production included a no-till drill for sowing cover crops, a tractor mounted cover crop roller (Bingham Brothers Inc., Lubbock, TX, USA), a tractor mounted rototiller, and a modified RJ tomato transplanter. For all the fungicide and insecticide applications, a JACTO vegetable air blast sprayer (Jacto Inc., Tualatin, OR, USA) mounted on a John Deere 4030 tractor (Moline, IL, USA) was used.

The interest on operating capital represents the opportunity costs of investing monies spent on variable costs in its next best alternative. This is calculated based using an interest rate of 7% over an investment period of six months (length of the tomato growing season). Overhead and management costs represent those costs that pertain to the operation of the whole farm that are partially attributed to the vegetable production enterprise, such as the costs for property taxes and insurance. Overall costs fluctuated between \$22,131 ha^{-1} to \$22,822 ha^{-1} due to changes in herbicide treatments and cover crop regimes.

Net revenue data, representing the return over total costs, was estimated by calculating total revenues for each plot on a per hectare basis and subtracting total costs. Only data from the Cullman, AL location was utilized for this analysis. Total crop revenue (\$ ha^{-1}) was calculated by multiplying the price of tomatoes (\$0.63 kg^{-1}) times the plot yield (kg ha^{-1}) [1]. Total costs were calculated using the cost budgets, adjusted for year (i.e. insecticide and fungicide costs). All estimates were calculated using 2005 dollars to minimize variability due to price fluctuations, allowing comparisons over time. Net revenue data was analyzed using analysis of variance as implemented in SAS® using PROC Mixed. Difference between treatments means were determined by single degree of freedom contrasts.

2. Results and discussion

2.1. Cover crop biomass

The quantity of cover crop biomass produced at both locations differed among cover crops, with rye producing 9363 kg ha^{-1}, and crimson clover producing 5481 kg ha^{-1} of dry matter. Turnip produced least biomass at 3860 kg ha^{-1}.

2.2. Weed control

The major weeds in the cover crop and plastic mulch plots included yellow nutsedge (*Cyperus esculentus* L.), smooth pigweed (*Amaranthus hybridus* L.), pokeweed (*Phytolaca americana* L.), tall morningglory [*Ipomoea purpurea* (L.) Roth], goosegrass [*Eleusine indica* (L.) Gaertn.], leafy spurge (*Euphorbia esula* L.), and broadleaf signalgrass [*Urochloa platyphylla* (Munro ex C. Wright) R.D. Webster] and ivyleaf morningglory (*Ipomoea hederacea* Jacq.). Other weed species included wild radish (*Raphanus raphanistrum* L.), Virginia buttonweed (*Diodia virginiana* L.), smallflower morningglory (*Jacquemontia tamnifolia* (L.) Griseb.). Weed control data for only the major weed species is discussed in this manuscript.

2.2.1. *Broadleaf signalgrass*

Broadleaf signalgrass was present only at Cullman in 2005. Averaged over ground cover treatments (**Table 1**), broadleaf signalgrass was controlled 11% without herbicides. Control improved significantly with herbicide application. *S*-metolachlor applied PRE controlled broadleaf signalgrass 79%; control improved to 97% when *S*-metolachlor PRE was followed by EPOST application of metribuzin fb LPOST clethodim application. Averaged over herbicide treatments (**Table 1**), turnip and crimson clover residue controlled broadleaf signalgrass 57% and 55% respectively. Control was significantly higher in rye and plastic mulch plots at 81% and 84% respectively compared to turnip and crimson clover plots.

Effect/ source	CYPES	AMAPA	DIGSA	BRAPP	ELEIN	PHTAM	PHBPU	EPHES	IPOHE	DIQVI	IAQTA	RAPRA
Environment (E)	0.401	0.044	<0.001	NA	NA	NA	NA	NA	NA	NA	NA	NA
Cover (C)	0.186	0.104	0.388	0.003	0.006	0.001	<0.001	<0.001	0.074	<0.001	<0.001	0.015
C × E	0.090	0.173	0.021	NA	NA	NA	NA	NA	NA	NA	NA	NA
Treatment (T)	0.021	0.006	<0.001	<0.001	<0.001	<0.001	<0.001	<0.001	0.496	0.157	0.058	<0.001
T × E	0.001	0.376	<0.001	NA	NA	NA	NA	NA	NA	NA	NA	NA
C × T	0.268	0.981	0.143	0.307	0.254	0.762	0.009	0.004	0.968	0.788	0.891	0.763
C × T × E	0.762	0.447	0.41	NA	NA	NA	NA	NA	NA	NA	NA	NA
Weeds were present in												
Year						Location						
2005	Cullman	Cullman		Cullman	Cullman	Cullman	Cullman	Cullman				
2006	Cullman	Cullman	Cullman						Cullman			
2006	Tuskegee	Tuskegee	Tuskegee							Tuskegee	Tuskegee	Tuskegee

CYPES, yellow nutsedge; AMAPA, palmer amaranth; DIGSA, large crabgrass; BRAPP, broadleaf signalgrass; ELEIN, goosegrass; PHTAM, pokeweed; PHBPU, tall morningglory; EPHES, leafy spurge; IPOHE, ivyleaf morningglory; DIQVI, virginia buttonweed; IAQTA, smallflower morningglory; RAPRA, wild radish.

Table 1. Analysis of variance for weed control[a].

2.2.2. *Goosegrass*

Goosegrass was present only at Cullman 2005. Averaged over all ground cover treatments (**Table 1**), goosegrass could not be controlled (6%) without herbicides. *S*-metolachlor PRE controlled goosegrass 76%. *S*-metolachlor PRE fb metribuzin EPOST fb clethodim LPOST controlled goosegrass 96%. Averaged over herbicide treatments (**Table 1**), turnip and crimson clover residue controlled goosegrass ≤ 60%. Rye residue and plastic mulch provided similar (80% and 79%) and higher control than turnip and crimson clover.

2.2.3. *Pokeweed*

Pokeweed was present at Cullman 2005. Averaged over ground cover treatments (**Table 1**) pokeweed was controlled 16% without herbicides. Control improved significantly with *S*-metolachlor PRE at 60% and *S*-metolachlor PRE fb metribuzin EPOST fb clethodim LPOST at 83%. Averaged over herbicide treatments (**Table 1**), turnip and crimson clover residue controlled pokeweed ≤ 40%. Rye residue controlled pokeweed 68% whereas pokeweed control was 86% in plastic mulch plots. However, the differences were not significant (P = 0.324) for rye and plastic mulch plots.

2.2.4. *Smooth pigweed*

Smooth pigweed was present at Cullman site during both the years. Averaged over ground cover treatments (**Table 2**), similar to other aforementioned weeds, smooth pigweed was controlled 9% in 2005 and 50% in 2006. None of the herbicide treatments provided acceptable control of smooth pigweed (≤70%). Averaged over herbicide treatments (**Table 1**) control was in general less in 2005 compared to 2006. Turnip residue suppressed smooth pigweed 30% in 2005 and 67% in 2006. Smooth pigweed was controlled 12% in 2005 and 52% in 2006 in crimson clover plots. Control was better in plastic mulch plots in 2005 (73%) but trend reversed in 2006, where rye plots recorded 71% and plastic mulch plots provided 57% control of smooth pigweed. However, differences in smooth pigweed control in rye and plastic mulch plots were not significant in either year.

Herbicide treatments		**Cullman 2005**				**Cullman 2006**			**Tuskegee 2006**						
Preemergence	Postemergence	BRAPP	ELEIN	PHTAM	AMACH	CYPES	AMACH	CYPES	DIGSA	IPOHE	CYPES	DIGSA	DIQVI	JAQTA	RAPRA
		%													
None	None	11	6	16	9	30	50	80	73	76	84	6	64	82	13
S-metolachlor	None	79	76	60	43	84	65	89	90	88	68	28	48	51	9
S-metolachlor	metribuzin fb clethodim	97	96	83	69	95	70	83	81	81	77	90	36	56	59
P-values from contrasts:															
PRE + POST *vs*.PRE alone		0.002	0.002	0.110	0.141	0.183	0.958	0.800	0.624	0.781	0.837	<0.001	0.761	0.949	0.003
PRE + POST *vs*. non treated		<0.001	<0.001	<0.001	<0.001	<0.001	0.546	0.973	0.793	0.907	0.856	<0.001	0.214	0.184	0.006
PRE alone *vs*. non treated		<0.001	<0.001	0.013	0.098	<0.001	0.717	0.682	0.284	0.539	0.510	0.133	0.587	0.103	0.965

Information about herbicide rate and application timing can be found in **Table 5**.

Table 2. Effect of herbicide treatments on broadleaf signalgrass (BRAPP), goosegrass (EELEIN), pokeweed (PHTAM), smooth pigweed (AMACH), and yellow nutsedge (CYPES), largecrabgrass (DIGSA), Virginia buttonweed (DIQVI), smallflower morningglory (JAQTA), and wild radish (RAPRA) control at Cullman and Tuskegee AL.

2.2.5. Yellow nutsedge

Yellow nutsedge was present at all the site years in this experiment. Averaged over ground cover treatments (**Table 1**), *S*-metolachlor applied PRE controlled yellow nutsedge only 55%. Bangarwa et al., have also reported less than 70% control of yellow nutsedge with S-metolachlor applied PRE in transplanted tomato in polyethylene mulch. Yellow nutsedge control increased to 70% when *S*-metolachlor was fb metribuzin EPOST fb clethodim LPOST. Averaged over herbicides rye residue provided 60% and Polyethylene mulch 65% control of yellow nutsedge.

2.2.6. Ivyleaf morningglory

Ivyleaf morningglory control did not differ among herbicide treatments. Averaged over herbicide treatments (**Table 1**), turnip and rye residue provided 94% and 90% control of ivyleaf morningglory. Control was 66% in crimson clover plots and 70% in plastic mulch plots.

2.2.7. Large crabgrass

No significant differences in large crabgrass control were observed among herbicide treatments. Averaged over herbicide treatments (**Table 1**) large crabgrass control was 88% in both turnip and rye plots. Control was 75% in crimson clover and plastic mulch plots.

2.2.8. Tall morningglory

Ground cover by herbicide treatment interaction was significant for tall morningglory control (**Table 3**). Ground cover treatments failed to control tall morningglory without herbicides (0–23%). Application of S-metolachlor controlled tall morningglory 41% in turnip plots but no control was observed in crimson clover plots. However, the same treatment provided good control of tall morningglory in plastic mulch (94%) and rye residue (98%) plots. S-metolachlor PRE fb metribuzin EPOST fb clethodim LPOST controlled tall morningglory ≤ 50% in turnip and crimson clover plots but controlled tall morningglory 98% in plastic mulch plots. Tall morningglory control declined to 71% in rye residue plots when S-metolachlor PRE was fb metribuzin EPOST fb clethodim LPOST.

Ground cover	Turnip	Turnip	Turnip	Clover	Clover	Clover	Plastic	Plastic	Plastic	Rye	Rye	Rye
Herbicide treatment	None	Pre	Pre + Post	None	Pre	Pre + Post	None	Pre	Pre + Post	None	Pre	Pre + Post
Variable costs												
Seeds/plants	984	984	984	896	896	896	838	838	838	887	887	887
Fertilizer	295	295	295	228	228	228	228	228	228	295	295	295
Herbicides	16	68	109	16	68	109	0	68	109	16	68	109
Insecticides	182	182	182	182	182	182	182	182	182	182	182	182
Fungicides	232	232	232	232	232	232	232	232	232	232	232	232
Scouting/soil tests	19	19	19	19	19	19	19	19	19	19	19	19
Custom harvest/grade/pack	7888	7888	7888	7888	7888	7888	7888	7888	7888	7888	7888	7888
Supplies (stakes, buckets, etc.)	6719	6719	6719	6719	6719	6719	6719	6719	6719	6719	6719	6719
Irrigation[b]	26	26	26	26	26	26	26	26	26	26	26	26
Machinery[c]	658	660	665	637	640	644	608	610	615	658	661	665
Labor[d]	559	565	575	550	555	565	1159	1164	1174	559	565	575
Interest on operating capital[e]	571	573	575	565	567	569	582	584	586	568	570	572
Total variable costs	18,150	18,211	18,268	17,958	18,019	18,076	18,480	18,558	18,615	18,050	18,111	18,168
Fixed costs												
Machinery[c]	1085	1090	1101	1026	1032	1043	998	1003	1014	1084	1090	1101
Irrigation[b]	1890	1890	1890	1890	1890	1890	1890	1890	1890	1890	1890	1890
Overhead/management[f]	1271	1275	1279	1257	1261	1265	1294	1299	1303	1264	1268	1272
Total fixed costs	4245	4255	4270	4173	4183	4198	4181	4192	4207	4238	4248	4263
Total costs	22,395	22,466	22,538	22,131	22,202	22,274	22,661	22,750	22,822	22,288	22,359	22,431

Note: Information about herbicide rate and application timing can be found in **Table 5**.
Source: Costs were based on cost estimates from Mississippi State (2005).
[a] The following assumptions were made in the estimation of the budgets: (i) plant 11960 plants ha^{-1}; (ii) fertigation was for 1 hr week^{-1}; (iii) 15.24 cm (6 in.) of water was applied during the growing season; and (iv) base yield was 39,230 kg ha^{-1} (35,000 lbs ac^{-1}). The yield assumption was needed for calculating harvesting/grading/packing costs.
[b] Variable irrigation costs represents expenditures for application of water during the growing season. Fixed irrigation costs represent the costs of the machinery for performing irrigation.
[c] Variable machinery costs represent costs for fuel, maintenance and repair. Fixed machinery costs represent the costs of purchasing the machinery, interest and depreciation.
[d] Labor costs represent the costs of operating machinery and hand labor during the growing season.
[e] The interest on operating capital represents the opportunity cost of investing the monies spent on variable costs into vegetable production.
[f] Overhead and management fixed costs represent overall farm management costs and general expenses for the whole farm that are partially applicable to the vegetable enterprises undertaken.

Table 3. Cost budgets (USD ha^{-1}) for tomato production by cover crop and herbicide treatment system at Cullman, AL, 2005[a].

2.2.9. *Leafy spurge*

Ground cover by herbicide treatment interaction was significant for leafy spurge also. Turnip and crimson clover residue failed to control leafy spurge with or without herbicides (**Table 3**).

Application of S-metolachlor alone controlled leafy spurge 86% in plastic mulch plots and 97% in rye residue plots. Control of leafy spurge increased in plastic mulch plots, when S-metolachlor PRE was fb metribuzin EPOST fb clethodim LPOST but decreased under rye residue.

This research demonstrates that high residue cover crops like rye can provide improved weed control compared to black polyethylene mulch. Crimson clover and turnip residue in general were less effective in controlling summer annual weeds. This could partially be due to less biomass production by these cover crops and also rapid decomposition of the legume residue due to lower C:N ratio. Decomposition rate of Brassicas is between grasses and legumes [31]. Another important factor which could have facilitated increased weed control by rye residue is rolling rye with mechanical roller crimper prior to its termination with glyphosate. The rolling process resulted in a uniform mat of residue on the soil surface that was a substantial physical barrier for weed seedlings to emerge through, compared to tomato plant openings in the plastic mulch system that provides no barrier. Despite improved weed control, herbicides were always required to provide acceptable weed control by ground cover treatments, which is in agreement with the previous research [16]. The PRE application alone was also not sufficient in controlling a majority of weeds. Yenish et al. [32] also reported inconsistent control with cover crop residue and concluded herbicides were always required to achieve optimum weed control in corn. However, Yenish et al. [32] cautioned weed control should not be the only criterion in selection of cover crops. Factors like cost and ease of establishment, impact on yield should be taken into consideration before selecting a cover crop.

2.3. Tomato stand establishment

No significant difference in stand establishment among the plastic mulch and rye residue plots. Crimson clover plots had fewer tomato plants compared to other treatments at Cullman 2005; however, the differences were not significant. Non-significant differences in tomato stand establishment were observed among ground cover treatments at Cullman 2006.

2.4. Tomato yield

Tomatoes were harvested only at the Cullman location in 2004 and 2005. There was no winter cover crop by herbicide interaction. Thus, the model reduces to a main effects model for winter cover crop and herbicide treatment effects. Tomato fruit yield was greater in 2005 compared to 2006. Pooled over herbicide treatments (**Table 4**), tomato yield was similar following rye cover and plastic mulch systems. Both these systems yielded 50 Mg ha^{-1} and 51 Mg ha^{-1} marketable tomato respectively in 2005, and 38 Mg ha^{-1} in 2006. However, the number of rotten tomato was more in plastic mulch plots than in rye plots in 2005, whereas no differences in total and marketable tomato yield were observed in these systems in 2006. Crimson clover plots yielded least in 2005. The lower yields following clover were likely due to higher weed interference in these systems. Yield was similar in turnip and crimson clover plots in 2006. Non-significant differences in tomato yield among ground cover treatments were observed in 2006. Averaged across ground cover treatments (**Table 2**), both herbicide regimen resulted in better yields compared to the no herbicide plots during both the years. Higher yields were obtained with the system containing both PRE and POST herbicide applications. Teasdale and Abdul-Baki [15] also concluded that marketable tomato yields were lower in cover crop treatments without herbicides than the corresponding treatments with herbicides in two of three years. No significant cover or herbicide treatment differences (P > 0.50) were observed for marketable classes of fruit, although there was a difference in frequency of market classes between the two years (data not shown). The number of small and medium-sized fruits was greater in 2005 than in 2006.

	Cullman					Cullman				Tuskegee				
	2005					2006				2006				
Cover	AMACH	BRAPP	CYPES	ELEIN	PHTAM	AMACH	CYPES	DIGSA	IPOHE	CYPES	DIGSA	DIQVI	JAQTA	RAPRA
	%													
Brassica	30	57	53	58	25	67	95	88	94	69	38	39	56	14
Crimson clover	12	55	70	50	38	52	69	75	66	80	39	54	71	9
Plastic	73	84	85	80	86	57	71	75	70	75	72	0	12	29
Rye	46	81	87	79	65	71	94	88	90	80	33	90	96	56
P-values from contrasts														
Brassica *vs*. Clover	0.770	0.998	0.591	0.886	0.904	0.916	0.219	0.726	0.139	0.992	1.000	0.864	0.860	0.992
Brassica *vs*. Plastic	0.050	0.023	0.043	0.107	0.002	0.970	0.234	0.719	0.190	0.820	0.014	0.301	0.190	0.820
Brassica *vs*. Rye	0.782	0.055	0.023	0.137	0.101	0.997	0.999	1.000	0.967	0.069	0.970	0.014	0.035	0.069
Clover *vs*. Plastic	0.005	0.016	0.446	0.017	0.009	0.997	1.000	1.000	0.995	0.663	0.016	0.069	0.038	0.663
Clover *vs*. Rye	0.243	0.036	0.302	0.023	0.348	0.817	0.263	0.735	0.277	0.038	0.957	0.084	0.180	0.038
Plastic vs. Rye	0.324	0.981	0.993	0.999	0.337	0.907	0.278	0.727	0.378	0.366	0.005	<0.001	<0.001	0.366

Information about herbicide rate and application timing can be found in **Table 5**.

Table 4. Effect of ground cover treatments on broadleaf signalgrass (BRAPP), goosegrass (EELEIN), pokeweed (PHTAM), smooth pigweed (AMACH) and yellow nutsedge (CYPES), ivyleaf morningglory (IPOHE), smallflower morningglory (JAQTA), and wild radish (RAPRA) control at Cullman and Tuskegee AL.

Preemergence[†]		Postemergence[‡]	
Herbicides	Rate (kg ha^{-1})	Herbicides	Rate (kg ha^{-1})
None	–	None	–
S-metolachlor	1.87	None	–
S-metolachlor	1.87	Metribuzin fb Clethodim	0.56 + 0.28

All preemergence herbicides were applied on the day of tomato transplanting
Postemergence application of metribuzin was accomplished 4 weeks after transplanting tomato followed by clethodim application at bloom initiation.

Table 5. Details of herbicide treatment rates and application timings.

		PHBPU				EPHES			
Herbicide treatments		Ground treatment				Ground treatment			
Preemergence	Postemergence	Turnip	Crimson clover	Plastic	Rye	Turnip	Crimson clover	Plastic	Rye
		%							
None	None	0	0	23	21	0	0	35	21
S-metolachlor	None	41	0	94	99	4	0	86	97
S-metolachlor	metribuzin fb clethodim	47	21	98	71	0	43	98	71
	P-values from contrasts								
PRE + POST *vs*.PRE alone		1.000	0.999	1.000	0.470	1.000	0.793	0.939	0.592

	PHBPU				EPHES			
PRE + POST *vs.* non treated	0.762	0.999	0.004	0.550	1.000	0.793	0.006	0.443
PRE alone *vs.* non treated	0.895	1.000	0.022	0.003	1.000	1.000	0.231	0.003

Information about herbicide rate and application timing can be found in **Table 5**.

Table 6. Effect of ground cover and herbicide treatments on tall morningglory (PHBPU) and leafy spurge (ESULA) control at Cullman, AL in 2005.

	2005	2006	2006	2005		2006	
Cover	Cullman		Tuskegee	Total	Marketable	Total	Marketable
	No. of Plants ha^{-1}			Mg ha^{-1}			
Brassica	10903	10671	8274	49	42	36	29
Crimson clover	9743	10980	6495	38	33	36	29
Plastic	12140	11135	6263	59	50	38	31
Rye	11522	11599	8351	58	51	38	31
P-values from contrasts							
Brassica *vs.* Clover	0.657	0.901	0.073	0.323	0.375	1.000	1.000
Brassica *vs.* Plastic	0.609	0.723	0.036	0.331	0.400	0.972	0.996
Brassica *vs.* Rye	0.926	0.180	1.000	0.462	0.348	0.970	0.998
Clover *vs.* Plastic	0.106	0.987	0.988	0.007	0.013	0.975	0.995
Clover *vs.* Rye	0.312	0.514	0.058	0.014	0.010	0.973	0.997
Plastic vs. Rye	0.926	0.723	0.027	0.996	1.000	1.000	1.000

Information about herbicide rate and application timing can be found in **Table 5**.

Table 7. Effect of ground cover treatments on tomato stand establishment at Cullman and Tuskegee AL and tomato yield at Cullman in 2005 and 2006.

		Cullman		Tuskegee	2005		2006	
Herbicide Treatments		2005	2006	2006	Total	Marketable	Total	Marketable
Preemergence	Postemergence	No of Plants ha^{-1}			Mg ha^{-1}			
None	None	11193	10381	6901	47	40	30	24
S-metolachlor	None	11019	11599	7365	50	42	40	33
S-metolachlor	metribuzin fb clethodim	11019	11309	7771	56	49	41	33
P-values from contrasts								
PRE + POST *vs.*PRE alone		1.000	0.730	0.789	0.452	0.366	0.991	0.997
PRE + POST *vs.* non treated		0.978	0.054	0.342	0.227	0.145	0.107	0.161
PRE alone *vs.* non treated		0.978	0.010	0.734	0.890	0.856	0.135	0.139

Information about herbicide rate and application timing can be found in **Table 5**.

Table 8. Effect of herbicide treatments on tomato stand establishment at Cullman and Tuskegee AL and yield at Cullman in 2005 and 2006.

Treatment		**Net Returns**		
Grond Cover	Herbicide	2005		2006
		USD ha^{-1}		
Turnip	None	7838	abc	-4199
Turnip	Pre	3461	ab	4654
Turnip	Pre + Post	6176	abc'	390

Treatment		Net Returns		
Crimson clover	None	−765	ab	566
Crimson clover	Pre	−1067	ab	−1274
Crimson clover	Pre + Post	8288	abc	2101
Plastic	None	9487	bc	−4884
Plastic	Pre	8720	abc	4563
Plastic	Pre + Post	9918	bc	2280
Rye	None	4060	abc	−190
Rye	Pre	13,924	c	341
Rye	Pre + Post	12,311	bc	1295

Single degree of freedom contrasts were conducted with SAS® PROC MIXED to examine differences between least square means at $P < 0.05$. Least square means followed by the same letter are not significantly different.

Table 9. Least square means of net returns over total costs for all the cover crop by herbicide systems at Cullman, AL. Information about herbicide rate and application timing can be found in **Table 5**.

2.5. Economic analysis

Economic costs of tomato production varied by treatment combination, but differences in costs due to treatment differences were relatively small overall, never larger than 3 percent of total costs (**Table 5**). Yield differences between treatments resulted in significant changes in total costs. Given that tomatoes were hand harvested, the cost of custom harvesting was the most significant cost of production (roughly 35 percent of total costs). Harvesting costs are a function of tomato yield. As yield increases, harvesting costs increase as more tomatoes need to be harvested from the field. Given that tomato yield varied significantly, this affected the total costs across treatments when calculating net returns. Furthermore, yield is a significant factor in calculating total crop revenue, resulting in significant variations in total crop revenue across treatments. Thus, primary differences in net revenue were primarily due to differences in tomato yields across treatments. However, given yield impacts both costs and revenues, net returns may not move in the same direction as yield.

In 2005, for all cover crop by herbicide system interactions, rye receiving only a PRE application provided the highest returns (\$13,924 ha^{-1}) followed by rye receiving both herbicide applications (\$12,211 ha^{-1}) (**Table 5**). The lowest returns in 2005 were from clover with only a PRE application (−\$1067 ha^{-1}) followed by clover with no herbicide application (−\$765 ha^{-1}). Both treatments with the highest return were significantly different from the two treatments with the lowest returns in 2005. For all the treatment combinations in between, excluding turnips with a PRE application, treatment differences were insignificant. In addition, results in 2005 indicate that there is no significant difference between using a rye cover crop or plastic under any of the alternative herbicide treatment regimes.

In 2006, the returns in general were significantly lower compared to 2005. In addition, differences in net returns between treatment combinations were not statistically significant (**Table 5**). The highest net returns were from using turnips with only a PRE application (\$4654 ha^{-1}), followed by plastic with only a PRE application (\$4563 ha^{-1}). Clover and rye returns were maximized when both PRE and POST herbicide application were applied. For the herbicide treatments, the highest returns were achieved with only the PRE emergence application and lowest when herbicides were excluded.

Our study indicates that winter cover crop residue can provide early season weed control with supplemental use of EPOST herbicides. However, total reliance on a winter cover crop for weed control was not sufficient, and in all cases herbicides were required to provide season-long weed control to maintain tomato yield. As hypothesized, it was evident that the use of winter cover crop for weed control cannot completely replace herbicides. However, by reducing the use of PRE herbicides, growers can decrease the amount of pesticide introduced into the environment. Our results further indicate that performance of a rye winter cover crop was either equal or comparable to plastic mulch in controlling weeds and maintaining tomato yields, thus reducing the need for tillage and other seedbed preparation operations. Tomato establishment was also not affected by presence of high residue at the time of transplanting, which is a valid concern in high residue conservation tillage systems. These findings can further the development of sustainable farming systems.

Results in this paper are short term effects of converting from a conventional plastic mulch system to three high-residue conservation tillage systems. These results indicate the economic possibility of growing fresh market tomatoes utilizing a conservation tillage system while maintaining yields and economic returns. However, the long term impact of these systems on yield and profitability require further investigation.

Author details

Andrew J. Price[1*], Jessica Kelton[2] and Lina Sarunaite[3]

*Address all correspondence to: andrew.price@ars.usda.gov

1 United States Department of Agriculture, Agricultural Research Service, National Soil Dynamics Laboratory, Auburn, AL, USA

2 Auburn University, Auburn, AL, USA

3 Institute of Agriculture, Lithuanian Research Centre for Agriculture and Forestry, Lithuania

References

[1] United States Department of Agriculture (USDA). 2008. Background Statistics: Fresh-market Tomatoes. http://www.ers.usda.gov/News/tomatocoverage.htm. Accessed: June 26, 2008.

[2] Blough, R.F., A.R. Jarrett, J.M. Hamlett, and M.D. Shaw. 1990. Runoff and erosion rater from silt, conventional, and chisel tillage under simulated rainfall. Transactions of ASAE. 33:1557–1562.

[3] Franzluebbers, A.J., G.W. Langdale, and H.H. Schomberg. 1999. Soil carbon, nitrogen, and aggregation in response to type and frequency of tillage. Soil Sci. Soc. Am. J. 63:349–355.

[4] Mahboubi, A.A., R. Lal, and N.R. Faussey. 1993. Twenty-eight years of tillage effects on two soils in Ohio. Soil Sci. Soc. Am. J. 57:506–512.

[5] Teasdale, J.R. and A.A. Abdul-Baki. 1995. Soil temperature and tomato growth associated with black polythene and hairy vetch mulches. J. Amer. Soc. Hort. Sci. 120:848–853.

[6] Abdul-Baki, A.A., J.R. Teasdale, R. Korcak, D.J. Chitwood, and R.N. Huettel. 1996. Fresh-market tomato production in a low-input alternative system using cover crop mulch. HortScience. 31:65–69.

[7] Teasdale, J.R. and A.A. Abdul-Baki. 1997. Growth analysis of tomatoes in black plastic and hairy vetch production systems. Hortscience. 32:659–663.

[8] Arnold, G.L., M.W. Luckenbach, and M.A. Unger. 2004. Runoff from tomato cultivation in the estuarine environment: biological effects of farm management practices. J. Exp. Marine Biol. Ecol. 2:323–346.

[9] Derpsch, R., C.H. Roth, N. Sidiras, and U. Köpke. 1991. Controle da erosão no Paraná, Brazil: Sistemas de cobertura do solo, plantio directo e prepare conservacionista do solo. Deutsche Gesellschaft für Technische Zusammenarbeit.

[10] Reeves, D.W. 2003. A Brazilian model for no-tillage cotton production adapted to the southeastern USA. Proc. II World Congress on Conservation Agriculture – Producing in Harmony with Nature. Iguassu Falls, Paraná, Brazil, Aug 11–15, 2003, pp. 372–374.

[11] Price, A.J., D.W. Reeves, and M.G. Patterson. 2006. Evaluation of weed control provided by three winter cereals in conservation-tillage soybean. Renewable Agric. Food Systems. 21:159–164.

[12] Reeves, D.W., A.J. Price, and M.G. Patterson. 2005. Evaluation of three winter cereals for weed control in conservation-tillage nontransgenic cotton. Weed Technol. 19:731–736.

[13] Sainju, U.M. and B.P. Singh. 2001. Tillage, cover crop, and kill-planting date effects on corn yield and soil nitrogen. Agron. J. 93:878–886

[14] Sainju, U.M., B.P. Singh, and W.F. Whitehead. 2002. Long-term effects of tillage, cover crops, and nitrogen fertilization on organic carbon and nitrogen concentrations in sandy loam soils in Georgia, USA. Soil Till. Res. 63:167–179.

[15] Arriaga, F.J. and K.S. Balkcom. 2006. Benefits of conservation tillage on rainfall and water management. In: Hatcher, K.J., editor. Proceedings of the 2005 Georgia Water Resources Conference, April 25–27, 2005.

[16] Teasdale, J.R. and A.A. Abdul-Baki. 1998. Comparison of mixtures vs. monocultures of cover crops for fresh-market tomato production with and without herbicide. Hortscience. 33:1163–1166.

[17] Creamer, N.G., M.A. Bennett, and B.R. Stinner. 1997. Evaluation of cover crop mixtures for use in vegetable production systems. HortScience. 32:866–870.

[18] Teasdale, J.R., C.E. Beste, and W.E. Potts. 1991. Response of weeds to tillage and cover crop residue. Weed Sci. 39:195–199.

[19] Saini, M., A.J. Price, and E. van Santen. 2006. Cover crop residue effects on early-season weed establishment in a conservation-tillage corn-cotton rotation. 28th Southern Conservat. Tillage Conf. 28:175–178.

[20] Teasdale, J.R. and C.L. Mohler. 2000. The quantitative relationship between weed emergence and the physical properties of mulches. Weed Sci. 48:385–392.

[21] Teasdale, J.R. 1996. Contribution of cover crops to weed management in sustainable agricultural systems. J. Prod. Agric. 9:475–479.

[22] Nagabhushana, G.G., A.D. Worsham, and J.P. Yenish. 2001. Allelopathic cover crops to reduce herbicide use in sustainable agricultural systems. Allelopathy J. 8:133–146.

[23] Teasdale, J.R. and C.S.T. Daughtry. 1993. Weed control by live and desiccated hairy vetch (*Vicia villosa*) . Weed Sci. 41:207–212.

[24] Abdul-Baki, A.A. and J.R. Teasdale. 1993. A no-tillage tomato Production system using hairy vetch and subterranean clover mulches. HortScience. 28:106–108.

[25] Abdul-Baki, A.A., J.R. Teasdale, R.W. Goth, and K.G. Haynes. 2002. Marketable yields of fresh-market tomatoes grown in plastic and hairy vetch mulches. HortScience. 37:878–881.

[26] Akemo, M.C., M.A. Bennett, and E.E. Regnier. 2000. Tomato growth in spring-sown cover crops. HortScience. 35:843–848.

[27] Masiunas, J.B., L.A. Weston, and S.C. Weller. 1995. The impact of rye cover crops on weed populations in a tomato cropping system. Weed Sci. 43:318–323.

[28] Price A.J., M.E. Stoll, J.S. Bergtold, F.J. Arriaga, K.S. Balkcom, T.S. Kornecki, and R.L. Raper. 2008. Effect of cover crop extracts on cotton and radish radicle elongation. Comm. Biometry Crop Sci. 3:60–66.

[29] Barnes, J.P. and A.R. Putnam. 1983. Rye residues contribute weed control in no-tillage cropping systems. J. Chem. Ecol. 9:1045–1057.

[30] Mississippi State Extension Service, Mississippi State University. 2005. Vegetable Planning budgets. http://msucares.com/pubs/infosheets/is1514.pdf. Accessed: July 29, 2008.

[31] Sustainable Agriculture Network. 2007. Managing Cover Crops Profitably, 3rd Edition. Sustainable Agriculture Network Handbook Series, Book 9. p. 73. Sustainable Agriculture Network, Beltsville, MD.

[32] Yenish, J.P., A.D. Worsham, and A.C. York. 1996. Cover crops for herbicide replacement in no-tillage corn (*Zea mays*). Weed Technol. 10:815–821.